PRAISE FOR CAL OREY
AND HER BELOVED HEALTH Ь

The Healing Powers of Tea

"Tea is an ancient elixir that is making quite a therapeutic come-back. I know this book will be your cup of tea!"
—Ann Louise Gittleman, Ph.D., C.N.S., author of *The Fat Flush Plan*

"*The Healing Powers of Tea*, like the drink itself, is a nourishing comfort."
—Dr. Will Clower, CEO Mediterranean Wellness

The Healing Powers of Vinegar

"A practical, health-oriented book that everyone who wants to stay healthy and live longer should read."
—Patricia Bragg, N.D., Ph.D., author of *Apple Cider Vinegar*

"Deserves to be included in everybody's kitchen and medicine chest."
—Ann Louise Gittleman, Ph.D., C.N.S., author of *The Fat Flush Plan*

"Wonderfully useful for everyone interested in health."
—Elson M. Haas, M.D., author of
Staying Healthy with Nutrition, 21st Century Edition

The Healing Powers of Olive Oil, Revised and Updated

"One of the most healing foods on the planet. A fascinating read—olive oil is not only delicious—it is good medicine!"
—Ann Louise Gittleman, Ph.D., C.N.S., author of
The Fat Flush Plan

"Orey gives kudos to olive oil—and people of all ages will benefit from her words of wisdom."
—Dr. Will Clower, CEO, Mediterranean Wellness

"Olive oil has been known for centuries to have healing powers and now we know why. It is rich in monounsaturated fats similar to avo-cado and macadamia nut oils. The information in this book will help you to understand the healing powers of oils."
—Fred Pescatore, M.D., M.P.H., author of *The Hamptons Diet*

The Healing Powers of Coffee

"A cup or two of joe every day is a good way to boost mood, energy, and overall health."
—Julian Whitaker, M.D., founder of the
Whitaker Wellness Institute

"For heart, mind, and body, Cal Orey shows us why coffee is the most comforting health food on the planet."
—Will Clower, Ph.D., CEO, Mediterranean Wellness

The Healing Powers of Honey

"A fascinating read about a natural remedy that is a rich source of antioxidants."
—Ray Sahelian, M.D., author of *Mind Boosters*

"Not everyone can be a beekeeper, but Cal Orey shares the secrets that honeybees and their keepers have always known. Honey is good for body and soul."
—Kim Flottum, editor of *Bee Culture* magazine and
author of several honeybee books

The Healing Powers of Chocolate

"The right kind, the right amount of chocolate may just save your life."
—Ann Louise Gittleman, Ph.D., C.N.S., author of
The Fat Flush Plan

"Chocolate is a taste of divine ecstasy on Earth. It is our sensual communion. Orey's journalistic style and efforts share this insight with readers around the world."
—Jim Walsh, founder of Intentional Chocolate

The
HEALING
POWERS
of TEA

Books by Cal Orey*

The Healing Powers of Tea
The Healing Powers of Vinegar
The Healing Powers of Olive Oil
The Healing Powers of Chocolate
The Healing Powers of Honey
The Healing Powers of Coffee

Doctors' Orders
202 Pets' Peeves

*Available from Kensington Publishing Corporation

The HEALING POWERS of TEA

CAL OREY

A COMPLETE GUIDE TO NATURE'S SPECIAL REMEDY

CITADEL PRESS
Kensington Publishing Corp.
www.kensingtonbooks.com

CITADEL PRESS BOOKS are published by
Kensington Publishing Corp
119 West 40th Street
New York, NY 10018

eISBN-13: 978-0-8065-3827-3
eISBN-10: 0-8065-3827-9
Kensington Electronic Edition: January 2018

ISBN-13: 978-0-8065-3826-6
ISBN-10: 0-8065-3826-0
First Citadel Trade Paperback Edition: January 2018

10 9 8 7 6 5 4 3 2 1

Printed in the United States of America

A special word of gratitude to my cat, Zen, and dog, Skyler, two beloved constants in my life—like hot or iced tea in the afternoon, night, and each season. Tea takes me to a special place I love. I cannot imagine my world without a cuppa. It would be like losing a best friend.

CONTENTS

Foreword

SWEET TEA: THE TABLE WINE OF THE SOUTH

Growing up in Alabama, I was that kid you couldn't keep inside, clean behind the ears, or out of the woods back behind our house. So I completely understand my mom signing her irrepressibly active son up for whatever sports might wear him out just a bit. Baseball was our favorite sport and, before each game, we had a ritual. We'd go to the "health food store" and buy a tiger's milk bar, which was supposed to give me energy (like I needed to be more kinetic) for the game. Looking back on it with a nutritionist eye, this was a nice idea, very well-intentioned but, because of its bizarre ingredients, at best irrelevant and at worst harmful.

It turns out that I was already consuming exactly what I needed to, almost every day. I needed no tigers, and certainly none of their milk.

In fact, like everyone else there we normally drank the table wine of the South, iced tea. It was just what you served for dinner (aka lunch) and supper (the evening meal), along with a squeeze of lemon and about two buckets of sugar per gracious glass. By the way, for us tea *is* sweet tea. And if you come down and ask for unsweetened tea, well y'all ain't from round here, are you?

What my mom didn't know was that tea has the particular kind of polyphenols called catechins and epicatechins that are amazingly healthy for you. These same catechins can increase blood flow to the muscles to increase the energy-producing mitochondria, and therefore overall energy levels. In other words, I was getting all the long-term benefits I needed right along with my collards, snap beans, and corn bread.

Of course, we didn't recognize this incredible health drink because the science wasn't as available as it is today, but also because it was so ordinary. It was just what we had every day. And in a world where TV scenes change every seven seconds and fads are expected to come and go until the next shiny bauble distracts our multitasking ADD brains to chase the puppy tail of the newest new miracle product, tea was for us a constant friend.

This was not true for only us, but actually for everyone on Earth. I wasn't surprised to learn that tea is the most consumed drink on the planet after water. It has been the expression of almost every culture to drink tea since we have been writing down what we eat and drink.

Not only is this drink easy to find, it's also dirt-simple to prepare. Just put leaves in a vessel of some kind, add hot water, and *voilà*, good tea! The same thing happens when you take coffee beans and add hot water—this "tea" of the beans becomes the incredibly healthful drink, coffee. The process of steeping these leaves and beans in hot water is so simple to do that it can be done at any time, right in your own kitchen.

Being so affordable, ubiquitous, and simple to prepare belies the fact that its everyday nature can make us look through, around, and over it. After all, how many times can you let people know that tea is amazing for a hundred reasons before they get distracted, then haul off and buy an abs buster and an energy drink to wash down their power bar?

That is why I'm personally very excited to see Cal's latest work in the *Healing Powers* series, because tea in every form is one of the most commonly available health items you can take. And while green tea has gotten a great deal of well-deserved attention, this book pulls in so much more in the white teas, black teas, and herbals that also have healing properties. The bottom line is that tea has been enjoyed by millions for millennia. And now *The Healing Powers of Tea* helps us better understand the full breadth of its wonderful healthful properties.

—Will Clower, Ph.D.
CEO, Mediterranean Wellness
Author of *The Fat Fallacy* and *The French Don't Diet Plan*

Preface

On a pre-winter day, I was sipping a cup of flavored black tea and enjoying the morning as a storm was brewing. I received an e-mail from my book editor. After almost two decades the message I awaited arrived. I got the go-ahead to write the tea *Healing Powers* series book. During the typing of my response, a large thump hit my cabin. I wrote, "I think we had an earthquake." The house shook again. I ran out into the living room. A pine tree was facing me outside the living room window—but it was horizontal not vertical on the deck. After I made a phone call to authorities, within an hour, the fire department, police, and building contractor were outside to see the damage. Wires were dangling everywhere outdoors. And my nerves were frazzled despite being a native Californian living in the mountains and used to storms and shakers.

I said, "Is it safe to make a cup of tea?" I repeated my words. Truly, I craved a cup of chamomile tea to comfort me so I could cope with the drama of the imperfect storm. One cup later: The power was out. On the upside, I landed the project: *The Healing Powers of Tea*—and I must tell you I feel this assignment had my name on it. It was fate.

During the creation of *The Healing Powers of Honey*, I wrote a chapter on teas to pair with honey varietals. Later, when I was a guest on national radio programs and at bookstore lectures and signings, I was asked, "What's the topic of your next book?" Without hesitation I answered, "Tea." What else could partner with books about chocolate and honey, right? So I put the idea on the back burner, year after year. And finally, the topic of tea whistled—and I'm glad it did. Despite the West Coast winter storm and falling tree, nothing was going to stop me now. I accepted the project and considered it an early holiday gift.

Born and raised in California, I'd love to tell you that I was a devout tea lover since I was a kid. It didn't happen that way exactly—but it did happen. As a post-hippie girl growing up amid the granola and tofu seventies, I ended up surrounded by tea—many types—and non-teas—the healing herbal ones. By being a Golden State native (a popular home of health nuts who will walk a mile or more for nature's finest tea), I won the key to enter Tea World—and I sense I am the author to do it right.

No, I am not a tea master who travels to India and China to get a face-to-face with the first flush of a specialty tea, nor a household-name doctor. But my credentials as a passionate author who writes for a mainstream audience (all ages) and a veteran health-nutrition journalist go back three decades. I've penned thousands of articles and more than a dozen books (big and small) on holistic-conventional remedies to nourish the body, mind, and spirit. And now, I'm taking you along with me on my past lifetime journey to a new place—into the land of tea. Yes, I am the down-to-earth West Coast author who is going to share with you both personal experiences and medical information on black tea and white tea—and herbal teas a part of the Mediterranean diet and lifestyle (an underlying theme in the *Healing Powers* series).

Like vinegar, olive oil, chocolate, honey, and coffee, tea is derived from nature. The five books in the *Healing Powers* collection all tout health benefits from these disease-fighting, antioxidant-rich foods, from ancient folk medicine to modern miracle. And now tea is going to join these superfoods.

So, like a tea plant plucker, I began my journey to a place I wanted to go to and the time is right for me to enter the world of tea. I am aware of the myriad of tea books but this story is unique because it's *my* up close and personal stories as a down-to-earth West Coast author on-the-road through decades of experiencing teas to tisanes. I will share with you my one-of-a-kind experiences delving into tea by tea and non-teas teamed with my travels out in the field and at home in Northern California. Once again, I find myself sitting in my mountain cabin by the lake writing a book.

So, I'll turn on the stove and heat water in the kettle, pour it into the white ceramic pot, and drink a cup of black tea in preparation to write the words I've wanted to share with you for a long, long time. Oh, and tea muffins are baking in the oven. In *The Healing Powers of Tea* I'll show you exactly how and why Tea World is a place I love to visit and I want to reveal my tea wisdom penned in "Cal-ese" with you and yours for your health's sake now and for years to come.

Acknowledgments

As a kid, I entered the land of tea not knowing how vast it is around the globe. As I grew up and began traveling across America with my dog, I met people and saw places where tea was a part of their lives—and I thank everyone and every place for the life-changing experiences.

Today, in the 21st century as the author of the *Healing Powers* series, I would like to express my heartfelt thanks to my publishing team at Kensington, and my editor who gave me the long-awaited project *The Healing Powers of Tea*. (Michaela Hamilton once told me, "I'm not saying 'no'—just not yet.") And the right time finally arrived.

I want to thank the savvy tea masters and tea merchants; Tea U.S.A., and its president, Peter Goggi; tea authority James Norwood Pratt; researcher Joe Vinson, Ph.D.; Dr. Will Clower, CEO, Mediterranean Wellness; Cal-a-Vie Health Spa and the Fairmont Hotel Vancouver; tearooms; and all the tea people I've interviewed and met in my travels who believe in the powers of tea.

I give this book as a gift to millennials (a person who was born in the 1980s or 1990s) and baby boomers (a person born between 1946 and 1964) and other generations before and after. Tea and tisanes will be a forever friend for you because they offer nature's remedy to help heal the mind, body, and spirit for you and yours—a timeless, reader-friendly book to pass on to generation after generation.

I feel blessed to have been given the opportunity to share my tea ex-

periences on the road and at home in the mountains. A toast to all of
you who have been with me through this journey—it's a place that I
was meant to go and it's a book that was destined to be written by
me—a loyal tea-loving West Coast girl who always comes back to the
Golden State and her cup of tea.

Author's Note

This book is intended as a reference tool only. It does not give medical advice. Be sure to consult your doctor or the appropriate health-care professional before starting any new diet or exercise program.

Real recipes, tried and true: The recipes in this book have been tested by me, my family and friends, and/or veteran chefs, bakers, and tea masters. Changing ingredients or using different tea brands or kitchen methods may alter taste, texture, and presentation of a dish. Plus, culinary palates vary. So use your own judgment and follow your instincts and personal tastes when you create a tea drink, tea-infused dish, or any tea recipe.

In the tea home cures and recipes, honey, nature's remarkable nectar, is often used. WARNING: To avoid infant botulism, do not feed honey to a baby who is younger than one year.

Remember, less is more in sweet, decadent desserts (so monitor portion control). Many sweets in moderation do have nutritional merits especially when teamed with fresh fruit and/or a cup of tea.

PART 1

TEA TIME

CHAPTER

1

The Power of Tea

*There are few hours in life more agreeable
than the hour dedicated to the ceremony
known as afternoon tea.*
—Henry James, *The Portrait of a Lady*

Every Sunday afternoon in our Kenton, England, estate at 4:00 P.M., like clockwork my mother would sigh, "It's time for a nice cup of tea." Then, she followed the routine like her grandmother did. She ordered tea and treats to her bedroom chamber. The parlor maid served us assorted crustless finger sandwiches, warm butter scones with Devonshire cream on a three-tiered tray, and we used a fancy British tea set. As we sipped brew from elegant white teacups, we talked about novels and travel. I was taught proper manners—from putting the white cloth napkin on my lap to keeping my elbows off the round table with white roses and vanilla-scented candles fit for royalty.

While this noble setting is a place I can picture me each afternoon, it is stretching the truth a tad. My real roots were not majestic or regal. There wasn't a castle or English servants, or chitchat like at the mad tea party in *Alice in Wonderland* or the tea gathering on the ceiling in *Mary Poppins*.

But there was tea in my early years, sort of. I grew up as the middle child of three in middle-class suburbia, San Jose, California. It was a mediocre place where my parents worked five days a week. A red and yellow Lipton Tea box was a staple in the kitchen cupboard. Iced tea in tall glasses with lemon slices was a commonplace on the wooden picnic table in the backyard in the summertime; hot tea with cinnamon sticks in copper mugs was a winter afternoon delight. A pretty lady in the newspaper ads and on the TV told me tea bags were for energy and relaxation; I believed her. And I recall in kindergarten singing the popular 20th-century song "I'm a Little Teapot, Short and Stout."

Now, in the 21st century, I can look back at my life experiences and see how tea—all types, one by one—played a role in my real world, then and now. True, I wasn't raised in a castle, nor as a kid did I engage in traditional afternoon tea. But I got a taste of tea—and non-teas or tisanes (a French word)—and its healing powers throughout my years of growing up and traveling on the West Coast, up to the Pacific Northwest, through the Midwest, the Gulf states, the Northeast, and Canada.

As I sit here in a rustic mountain cabin surrounded by pine trees (recalling the one that fell on the roof when I landed this tea book project), I feel a connection with tea leaves—and flowers, roots, and bark as I write *The Healing Powers of Tea*. My cupboards are stuffed with tea and non-tea types: in decorative tea tins, big and small, and a big Lipton box, too, like when I was a kid. The best part, I have discovered the healing magic of tea is a big place—and I've done my homework to dish on teas and non-teas that I love and to help you discover your tea love.

For countless people—and perhaps for you, too—the healing powers of tea are no secret. Like me, people use tea not only as a versatile home cure for ailments but also as a weight loss, heart-healthy, cancer-fighting, and anti-aging superfood, where it gives a health boost teaming up with clean foods, including fruits, herbs and spices, and water. But people also love a cup of tea because of its flavor and feel-good vibe.

If you haven't heard by now, listen up. Your health—mind, body, and spirit—may depend on it. Chances are, you already have one great tea folk remedy in your kitchen cupboard. It's time to start using it more. But there is another tea on the block that you need to know about, too.

Medical doctors and even tea researchers are now discovering just what folk herbalists around the world have been saying for centuries, that *both* black tea and white tea may have remarkable healing powers.

Today, we know more about the natural goodness behind these two teas. Both black and white tea are good folk medicine. And this healthful yin and yang duo (the Chinese principles of opposite and complementary elements to achieve harmony) promises to be more popular as a home remedy combination in the new millennium, as alternative medicine—which includes tea—continues to be used more and more. Studies have shown antioxidants (in superfoods, including black tea and white tea) act like pharmaceuticals, which are currently being researched for their potential to treat diseases and stall aging.

Tea, which is considered a superfood, is believed by medical authorities to help lower the risk of developing health ailments and diseases because it has the same compounds as antioxidant-rich staples. Researchers have connected diet with the prevention and treatment of cancer, diabetes, and heart disease. Tea studies on nonhumans as well as humans will most likely continue in the future as scientists seek to discover more healing powers of nature's special remedy.

THE BLACK AND WHITE TEA LEAF YIELD TWO POWERFUL TEAS

Black tea has been praised by wellness gurus as one of Mother Nature's most versatile superfoods, especially if produced from quality, organically grown tea plants. And now, white tea, the overlooked and under-studied tea, may be its new counterpart, thanks to the white tea leaves.

People from all walks of life—as well as some tea pioneers from past centuries and recent times and present-day medical researchers—agree energizing black tea (which goes through a longer process of oxidation than other tea varieties) first and foremost lowers the risk of heart disease and stroke.

Surprisingly, medical doctors and tea researchers continue to spread the word that *both* black tea and white tea may be the new green tea (or coffee) while their reputation of healing powers grows within the tea industry. While black tea (the most popular tea type in the United States) may also ward off inflammation linked to chronic conditions like cancer, diabetes, and aging, white tea isn't to be ignored. . . .

When it comes to preventing heart disease, stroke, and cancer, white tea may be just as powerful as green tea, if not more so. White tea (less processed and more antioxidants than black tea and green tea) may be the better choice of tea to stave off some health ailments and diseases. So, these two teas—black and white (and blends with both or either one)—are the up-and-coming surprising superstars in the land of tea.

> Tea: a drink that is made by soaking the dried leaves of an Asian plant in hot water
> —Merriam-Webster Dictionary

A TIME FOR TEAS AND TISANES

While it's my mission and passion to tout ancient and present-day findings about black tea and white tea, green tea, and other teas—tisanes are in the mix, too. As a popular remedy in ancient days, it is the time for tea in the 21st century. And not only are medical doctors, researchers, and tea advocates praising the merits of tea and tisanes; so are people in the limelight and everyday folks, too.

Dr. Mehmet Oz more than once on TV has discussed the powers of teas, including its weight loss potential that may work if used at different times of the day. Celebrity tea lines including Lady Gaga's and Padma Lakshmi's have touted the healing powers of tea, not to forget Oprah and her love for chai (a black tea with spices and milk). The consuming thirst for tea is hot and getting hotter for age-defying baby boomers, like me, and millennials who face the novelty of high-quality tea.

TEA FORMS TO TASTE

Like more than 50 percent of American households, you may have at least one type of tea in your kitchen cupboard, but there are a variety of forms of tea available for both your health and enjoyment, too. Here is a chart of four forms of commercial teas. It's advised by tea researcher Joe Vinson in the Chemistry Department, University of Scranton, Scranton, PA, to use tea from bags or loose leaves to get the most disease-fighting polyphenol antioxidants.[1]

Form	Description of Tea	Taste, Texture, Treats
Tea bags	Bags or sachets with tea leaves from the plant	Flavorful, clean, no leaves, convenient
Loose leaves	Contains leaves	Fresh, strong like coffee beans, tranquil ritual
Powder	Finely ground powder	Grainy if not blended, lacks freshness
Bottled	Ready-to-drink tea in bottles	Tasty, a wide variety, smooth, convenient, RTD tea boasts differentiated flavors

FROM PLANT LEAVES TO SUPER TEA

Not only are there different forms of tea to drink, but there are also a variety of teas (like antioxidant-rich chocolates and olive oils) touted by people—from foodies to tea enthusiasts—as one of Mother Nature's superfoods. And now, healing teas—not just black tea—are making news around the world, and are popular in restaurants, beauty spas, and in our homes.

Tea is not just a cooling beverage you drink iced in the summertime or hot beverage to warm you up in the wintertime. It's an ancient medicine that has been used to treat heart disease, respiratory ailments, skin ulcers, wounds, stomach problems, insomnia, and even "superbugs." Tea is also known to help curb sweet cravings and boost energy, which can help stave off type 2 diabetes, as well as unwanted pounds and body fat.

Top scientists, nutritionists, and medical doctors know stacks and stacks of research show some teas contain the same disease-fighting antioxidant compounds that are found in fruits and vegetables, which fight heart disease, cancers, diabetes, and obesity—four problems in the United States and around the world. Some of the medical doctors I interviewed in the early 21st century for my book *What 101 Doctors Do to Stay Healthy* (Kensington, 2002) touted the healing powers of tea (especially green tea) and shared personal experiences of how it helped to curb their appetite and to boost the immune system.

101 Miracle Foods That Heal Your Heart author Liz Applegate, Ph.D., like other doctors (and me) who praise superfoods, points out that *both* black and green tea help protect against heart disease. Drinking your tea hot or cold, regular or decaf, brewed or instant, can put you on the right track for your heart, notes Applegate. She's hardly alone about touting the variety of teas for tea time.[2]

Jonny Bowden, Ph.D., author of the timeless book *The 150 Healthiest Foods on Earth: The Surprising, Unbiased Truth About What You Should Eat and Why*—one of my go-to health books—also praises tea (black, white, green, and oolong). He concludes a section on tea with a subhead title "Everyone Benefits from Tea." He agrees with tea gurus, giving a lot of health credit to tea's antioxidant protection, which helps guard against heart disease *and* cancer.[3]

Most medical doctors I spoke with during my trek through Tea World agreed that tea is something to include on your superfood list—and that because of other health virtues you can reap, it should be your standout beverage of choice. Antioxidant guru Jeffrey Blumberg, Ph.D., of Tufts University tells it like it is: "In sum, tea is a natural, zero-calorie, flavonoid-rich, aromatic and delicious beverage with a 5,000-year history associated with health and wellness and a 20-year history of scientific substantiation of these benefits." He adds, "If Americans consumed more tea (of any color) and drank less sugar-sweetened beverages like soda, it would certainly reduce their risk of type 2 diabetes and heart disease." So, why are the antioxidants in tea so good for you, anyhow?

Health-Boosting Nutrients in Tea

Medical researchers around the world continue to find new health-promoting nutrients believed to be in tea. Most important, like red wine, green tea, and certain fruits and vegetables, tea contains antioxidants—disease-fighting enzymes that protect your body by trapping free-radical molecules. (Imagine video game–like bright silver sharks with mouths that open and close, swimming after big bad bugs and gobbling them up before any damage occurs to a human body.)

Past and ongoing medical research shows that consuming antioxidant-rich tea may lower the risk of developing heart disease, cancer, and even stall the aging process. Researchers continue to find new health-promoting nutrients in certain superfoods, and here are some of the super ones in tea that you should know about:

Catechin: a powerful polyphenol that acts as an antioxidant and can help strengthen immune responses

ECGC: Epigallocatechin-3-gallate is an antioxidant found in black, white, green, and oolong teas

Flavonoids: powerful disease fighters that may help to fight allergies, carcinogens, inflammation, and viruses

Flavanols and Flavonols: a group of plant compounds (from flavonoids, a large group of phytonutrients) found in some tea that have shown antioxidant effects which may help lower the risk of developing heart disease, some forms of cancer, and diabetes

L-theanine: an amino acid found in teas that provides a sense of relaxation and stress relief

Tannins: nutrients that may help inhibit plaque buildup that causes heart attacks and strokes

Polyphenols: natural compounds that act as powerful antioxidants that protect your body by trapping the free-radical molecules and getting rid of them before damage occurs

Theaflavins: antioxidant polyphenols found in black and green tea that may help lower the risk of heart disease and cancer because of their antiviral and anti-cancer effects

(*Sources: The Healing Powers* series; Tea Fact Sheet, Tea Association of the U.S.A., Inc.)

ALL TEA COMES FROM ONE PLANT

Okay. I confess at one time I believed that tea came from multiple colored trees: black, white, and green, like when Dorothy entered the land of Oz with its talking trees and vibrant colors. But in the real world of tea, black, white, green, oolong, and dark teas all come from the same plant, a warm-weather evergreen named *Camellia sinensis*. It's the harvesting and art of production and oxidation that differentiates one tea from another.

The following types of tea—some of the top antioxidant-rich and medicinal ones—are listed below from A to Z. These teas (bags and loose leaves) are sitting side by side in boxes and tin cans in my pantry. One by one, I encounter each flavor, and it's advised to use different teas to benefit from different healing powers. I use each one of them for a variety of reasons, including drinking, cooking, baking, beauty, and more. I dish out more details for you about the tea types in the following chapters and throughout *The Healing Powers of Tea*—but my focus is on black tea (common varieties and new findings), white tea (common varieties and new findings), red tea (and demystifying it), and popular tisanes.

Herbal teas or tisanes, unlike tea, come from a wide variety of flowers, trees, and plants. There are hundreds of varieties found around the world. There are so many herbal teas it's difficult to choose which ones are the best to write home about because the superstars with medicinal value deserve kudos for a variety of reasons. It's not unusual to blend tea types and teas with tisanes—it opens up a wide world of tea love. But first, let's delve a bit more into the number of tea types or varieties.

You may discover, like I did, that the categories of tea differ from four (major types) to five and six true teas. It doesn't seem like there is one answer that fits all. It depends on whom you ask, though. The Cozy Tea Cart tea master Danielle Beaudette, who lists six teas—black, dark, green, oolong, white, and yellow—explains, "The teas that fall under dark tea category used to be classified under black teas." Then, these teas were given their own category due to the aging process. Since yellow tea is rare—it's not often included in tea types lists—I focus on the four.

THE HEALING TEA PARADE

Type	Tea Color	Flavor and Scent
Black	Dark, reddish-black	Bold, strong, robust
Dark	Dark, black	Strong, earthy
Green	Light green, golden in color	Grassy
Oolong	Orange-red	A mix of bold and grassy; fruity aroma
White	Light yellow	Sweet, mellow
Yellow	Yellow	Sweet and savory

(*Source:* Tea Association of the U.S.A., Inc. Tea & Health: An Overview of Research on the Potential Health Benefits of Tea)

It's important to be aware of these tea types *and* the steeping temperature of your tea—black, white, and green—since it may affect the amount of antioxidants you get in your cup, reports the *Journal of Food Science*. Researchers found that antioxidants were affected by the time factor: Black tea provides the most antioxidants in a short hot water steeping; white tea, the longer time, the more antioxidants; and green tea showed longer steeping (two hours) produced the most antioxidants.[4]

SPECIALTY TEAS ARE SPECIAL

So, there is tea and there is more tea. Welcome to the sphere of good-for-you specialty teas. Specialty tea is defined as teas of special or high quality. But it's a bit more complicated when you dig deeper into the world of special(ty) teas. The term "specialty tea" can daze and confuse you when other words like "artisan," "fine," "gourmet," and "premium full-leaf teas" (handcrafted in limited amounts for a special person or time of year) come into play, making a simple definition of specialty tea not so simple or definitive.

Let me give you a breakdown of this intriguing category of teas that deserve special attention. Specialty teas are high-quality products from a variety of regions, harvests, varied blends, flavors, scents and/or single-origin estate teas—comparable to exceptional chocolate and coffee. But that's not all. . . .

Fine Teas: The Specialty Tea Institute (a division of the Tea Association of the U.S.A., Inc., and established in 2002) explains specialty teas are "like fine wines" and "have an almost infinity variety of flavors, origins and appearances, as well as a rich history and variety of traditions." That is a good and simplified start when explaining specialty tea, much like specialty chocolate, coffees, and olive oils. The different types remind me of the film *Scott Pilgrim vs. the World*, when Ramona offers him a dozen different kinds of tea, which can be mind-boggling to a novice tea drinker. But there's more . . .

A buzzworthy creation of fresh, expertly processed, high-end teas from exotic origins, either in loose leaf form or packed in sachets. Specialty tea is blossoming in popularity and is a "star" in the tea industry, according to the Tea Association of the U.S.A., Inc. The higher-end teas, like specialty teas, are forecasted to continue to be in the limelight and expand in the future.[5]

Tea Passion: Also, it's no surprise that progressive millennials are infatuated with progressive specialty teas and enjoy discovering new and distinguished flavors, ethnic or new cultural tea offerings, and craft selections. Specialty teas attract health-conscious people, from baby boomers indulging in the amazing natural health perks of different tea varieties to millennials who love to try exotic foods that can give them a sense of traveling to faraway lands.

Specialty Tea Institute member Danielle Beaudette, who sells high-quality teas (85 percent of her tea collection) and provides guided tours to tea estates in Sri Lanka and India, dishes a definition for the special teas. "Specialty tea is whole-leaf tea from the *Camellia sinensis* bush that is hand plucked by tea pluckers. The bushes are grown in elevations of 3000–8000 feet in clean, mountainous air." These words ring true but there is more to it when defining the specialty tea, especially for the housewife in Lexington, Kentucky, to the retired senior in Miami, Florida, or a tea-loving health-conscious author like me, and perhaps you, too. I still want more.

So *exactly* where does specialty tea come from and how do I know if I am purchasing it? Specialty teas include a wide group of extraordinary teas—unique in a variety of ways—so a hearty description is in order. Specialty teas may come from a specific region touted for its premium quality. Also, these special teas may come from a noteworthy tea garden or estate (similar to enthusiasts who go on the quest for special olive oil in the Golden State or to Europe).

Specialty Tea Samples Please: Specialty tea need not be unblended. The definition may also include teas that utilize traditional recipes, which are recognized within the industry as being of high quality. An example of this definition is an English Breakfast blend that tradition-ally uses high-quality, 100-percent China Keemun or a blend of Ceylon and India teas. Other examples of this type of specialty tea are blends called Irish Breakfast or Russian Caravan, a smooth black tea. In addition, flavored teas such as Earl Grey (flavored with oil of berg-amot), scented teas such as jasmine (a green tea flavored with jasmine flowers), spiced teas (flavored with ginger), and a tea that undergoes special processing such as a Lapsang souchong (which has a smoky fla-vor) are also referred to as specialty teas.

Savoring Special Teas: Specialty teas are available at tearooms, super-markets, and luxury health spas. Big and small tea companies can and do include signature house blends, single-estate teas, and rare teas as men-tioned earlier. Tea menus at tearooms show how specialty teas can be pricey. A sampling may be sobering, such as Geisha Blossom Tea $8: Elegant and highly refined blend of green tea; Kenilworth $10: A wonderful TWG Tea Ceylon tea; White Immortal Tea $21: Silver tips of Yin Zhen.

And the Vancouver, British Columbia, Fairmont Teas collection of-fered in their tearoom, for example, is impressive, including both black teas like Margaret's Hope Darjeeling, and white teas like White Monkey Paw, China. The menu offers a fine collection of unique teas and herbal teas, too. Sourced from China, India, Sri Lanka—and in-cluding herbal selections from Egypt and Italy. The specialty tea list includes green and oolong teas and herbal delights.

Flavored teas, such as Earl Grey, scented teas such as jasmine, and spiced teas can all fall under the umbrella term of specialty or artisan teas. Stash Tea and Teavana are just two big brands of dozens of brand names in the specialty tea segment.

Once you are treated to a tea collection, in a tearoom, on a tea es-tate, or in the comfort of your home, specialty teas will make it tough to go back to a mass-produced tea bag—but doable if you're surviving a natural disaster or suffering from jet lag. Just kidding. But when you drink a cup of special specialty tea it's time to enjoy because you're getting the crème of the crop. In the 21st century, black, white, oolong, green, and herbal specialty teas are easier to find than they were in the 1900s—not just in tearooms or tea shops—but in supermarkets and on major shopping Web sites, as well as individual shops online, too. And yes, this is good to know for both you and me.

10 TIDBITS TO SWEETEN THE TEAPOT

Now that you got more than a sip of the semantics of specialty tea, did you know humankind's relationship to the tea plant goes back to ancient days and is still part of our lives? We are connected because of the multifaceted usage of tea around the globe. It makes sense to dish out a heaping spoonful of tea leaf trivia to show you just how amazing the tea plant is to you and me. Take a look at these 10 factoids that'll get you thinking about how amazing Tea World actually is.

1. Tea leaves sprout at the top of the *Camellia sinensis* tea plant.
2. The "tea belt" is primarily in Asia, where it has a tropical or subtropical climate. Some leading tea-producing countries include Argentina, China, India, Indonesia, Japan, Kenya, Malawi, Sri Lanka, Tanzania, and Taiwan.
3. Tea producers in the United States include Alabama, Hawaii, South Carolina, and Washington. Herbal tea production is popular in the Pacific Northwest—Washington and Oregon.
4. There are more than 3,000 varieties of tea grown around the globe.
5. The United Sates is the third largest importer of tea in the world, after Russia and Pakistan.
6. Elevenses is a term for what happens at 11 o'clock A.M. in England; it's a tea break to enjoy a cup of tea and some cookies or cakes—to help you stay on the top of your game at work or play.
7. On any given day, more than half of the American population drinks tea . . .
8. The South and Northeast have the greatest concentration of tea drinkers.
9. Approximately 85 percent of tea consumed in America is iced.
10. It's advised to use good-tasting tap water, or filtered or bottled water.

(*Source:* Tea Association of the U.S.A., Inc.)

As you can see, tea (a functional food that boasts super health benefits) is enjoyed around the globe and is in demand. Some tea companies and medical researchers avoid dishing hype on the health virtues of tea because more research is needed, especially with some teas and tisanes. Many tea connoisseurs believe you should drink tea for enjoyment and relaxation. Also, others insist that drinking a variety of teas and tisanes is healthier than putting all of your tea leaves in one basket.

Bear in mind, no one tea—or too much of it—is a magic bullet cure-all for an ailment or disease. It's a combination of a healthy diet, clean lifestyle, good luck, and incorporating a variety of nature's special remedy into your day and night, year after year, that will give you the healing powers of tea.

LOVING A KETTLE AND A POT

Okay, okay. I confess that more times than I can count I'll fill a cup with tap water and place it into the microwave. Two minutes later, I'll dunk a tea bag into the water—and I am tagged a tea-bag dunker. But in my defense, I have mastered the art of brewing a pot of tea; it's a ritual that is well worth the time and effort.

I used an electric stainless steel kettle for the first time in a Vancouver, British Columbia, hotel room on the 29th floor with a "million-dollar view" of the English Bay and the North Shore Mountains. Sipping a cup of black tea (from a basic black tea bag) on the balcony was an unforgettable escape.

If you have a stainless steel kettle, you can begin with it. Start with fresh cold water—most tea proponents advise filtered water or bottled water. (I use fresh water from the tap.) Remove the lid and fill the kettle with the amount of cups of tea you'll be serving (two cups for two cups of brew). Replace lid and place on stovetop burner on medium heat. Chill until your kettle whistles. During this time rinse a ceramic teapot (a built-in infuser is convenient) with hot water to warm it up, which will help prevent any cracks. Add tea bags or loose leaves in the strainer. Remove tea kettle from stovetop burner and pour water into the teapot from the kettle. Allow the tea to steep. Also, rinse teacups in hot water to stave off any cracking. (Warning: Once you brew a pot of tea and use tea leaves, going back to tea bags and the microwave will seem like a mortal sin and guilt will set in.)

For cold-infused tea (any type of tea and fruits, herbs, spices), toss a few bags into a 2-quart pitcher (4 cups) of cold water. Cover and refrigerate for several hours. If you use loose leaf tea, put in 2 tablespoons per quart of water.

You now have Tea Basics 101 down. You also have a tea brewing method ready to use, so take a tea break. Here is a special recipe to whip up and savor with a cup of tea as you sit down, lie down, and cozy up. Come with me on an adventurous trip through Tea World. You can visit bit by bit, or all at once, and return again for a myriad of health reasons including rest and relaxation for your mind, body, and spirit.

Raisin Scones

Twice when I was visiting Vancouver, British Columbia, I was smitten by the warmth and airy ambiance of tearooms: fresh, warm scones with clotted cream and tea— genuine deliciousness. This recipe is straight from the prestigious Fairmont's chef and a place where I feel like a princess when sipping tea and savoring a fresh, warm scone.

WET INGREDIENTS

2 whole eggs (plus another one to brush scone tops)
1 cup whipping cream

Whisk eggs and cream together in a bowl and set aside.

DRY INGREDIENTS

¾ cup unsalted butter
¾ cup white sugar
3¼ cups baker flour

1 tablespoon baking powder
1 cup raisins

Sift all dry ingredients together in a bowl. Add the wet ingredients (whipping cream and eggs) with the dry ingredients (butter, sugar, flour, and baking powder) and mix just until moist. Add the raisins and slowly mix. Place dough on a floured surface and roll out. Cut either into rounds or triangles and brush the tops with a beaten egg. Place on a baking sheet and bake at 325 degrees for 15 to 20 minutes. Serve with Devon cream and jam and enjoy! Makes 15 scones.

(*Courtesy:* Executive Chef Cameron Ballendine of the Fairmont Hotel Vancouver)

In this book, I will show you how drinking tea with the Mediterranean-style healing superfoods is a healthy choice you can make every day. But many people, perhaps you, will not want to reap the benefits of *all* teas and/or some herbal teas by sipping the brew. So, you can get your daily tea dose from tea-infused cuisine, and use it in other remarkable ways, too. I've included dozens of recipes to pamper your penchant and to help heal your whole being, too.

But first, let's go way, way back into the past. Take a trip with me to discover the history behind tea and how it's one of the ancient world's first—and most amazing—natural medicines with healing powers.

TEA-CENTRIC HEALING HINTS TO STEEP

Research in the late 20th century and 21st century shows that quality teas from the tea plant, and tisanes, which are derived from a variety of flowers, bark, plants, and trees, produce a brew from around the globe—and may help you to:

✓ Stay heart-healthy and keep your blood pressure and cholesterol numbers in check.

✓ Enhance your immune system to fight off colds and flu.
✓ Lower your risk of developing cancer.
✓ Stave off diabetes.
✓ Treat respiratory diseases.
✓ Help you lose unwanted pounds and body fat.
✓ Add quality years to your life.

An Ancient Cuppa Comfort

But indeed, I would rather have nothing but tea.
—Jane Austen, *Mansfield Park*

My first real-life encounter with tea was when I was a preschooler in the safe suburbia of San Jose, California—a place for middle-class nuclear families in the fifties. Our neighborhood was a replica of normalcy: two parents, two point five children, one dog, a track home with manicured green lawns, the milkman and ice cream truck were our neighborhood excitement. One hot summer evening for the novelty factor I asked my mother if I could have a tea party.

She prepared a tray for "high tea" (or meat tea, the English name for the evening meal). Cold cuts (cheeses and meats), breads and jams, and a surprise tart—minus black tea (my parents drank it, but it was off-limits to kids because of the caffeine). I improvised. It was a spin-off of *Alice's Adventures in Wonderland*'s "A Mad Tea Party"—but I was the host clad in my pink Easter dress and pink bonnet.

In the clean and cool dining room, I set up a tablescape on our rectangle glass table (which I have now and cherish for my own tea occasions), complete with blue- and gold-flowered teacups and saucers, a matching teapot, cream and sugar bowls, and a tray. I invited my Dalmatian dog, Casey, and stuffed animals: a plush Russian Blue cat, Sapphire, and a fluffy white rabbit, Harvey.

"Welcome, my friends!" I exclaimed to my attentive four-legged trio. I poured water into dainty blue- and gold-flowered cups. Peanut butter and fruit jam sandwiches, animal crackers, and mini lemon curd tarts made my tea party an unforgettable ceremonial event that paved my way for enjoying nature's special brew and its healing powers.

My fantasy of drinking tea with humans in a tea garden setting as well as in a tearoom never disappeared throughout the wonder years of growing up. Not only did my first tea party (without the real beverage) amuse me—morning tea and tea late in the evening did come to me at the right time, right place.

The years passed, and once a teenager, I was served iced sweet tea with lemon and ice cubes in the springtime . . . and hot black tea with orange slices and cinnamon sticks in copper mugs during the fall. The scents of these drinks still linger in my mind, and ended up being the gateway for me into Tea World, a place more magical and mystical than I ever imagined.

The Story of Afternoon Tea

As the tale goes, the Duchess of Bedford was the royal woman behind a traditional ritual—"afternoon" or "low" tea. Evidently, one day in 1840, the noon meal did not satisfy the duchess, who felt under the weather late that afternoon. It is believed the duchess asked her servants to bring her a pot of tea and snacks. With a European air about the event, she invited friends to join her for an additional afternoon meal at five o'clock in her Belvoir Castle. The Tea Menu offered a variety of cakes, sandwiches, and assorted sweets—and tea. This ritual grew par for the course, so when the duchess went back to London, the custom was for her to invite friends for tea. The custom was well accepted and mimicked by other socialites and thus afternoon tea was born and lives on into the 21st century. Tea time—at all times of day and night—is today celebrated in our homes and in tearooms around the globe.

TEA AND ITS HISTORY

As history tells it, Chinese emperor Shen Nung, also called the "Divine Healer," is the man who deserves credit for discovering tea leaves and their versatile healing powers. The story goes that tea was discovered by this man back in 2737 BC. The emperor sensed that people who drank boiled water reaped the benefits of better health and well-being. Then, when tea leaves fell into his boiling water, Shen Nung was pleasantly surprised by the good aroma, and great flavor. After this unforgettable blessing in disguise, a cup of perfect tea was celebrated, and the finding was noted by people in China, Japan, and other faraway lands. And that is the story of how a cuppa tea got its roots, with thanks to a health-minded man of nobility who was at the right place at the right time. Cheers.[1]

The emperor may have been the first human to celebrate the benefits of tea, but he certainly was not the last. Back in the ancient past, the tea plant was noted for its versatile medicinal purposes, with benefits ranging from physical stamina to mental well-being. The healing powers of tea were put to work by Egyptian physicians as long as 5,000 years ago. In the Old World, tea was also used by practitioners of traditional Chinese medicine and religious travelers from Asia, the place of its roots.

The Buddhist Monk Wakes Up to Tea

Back in early 500s to 600s CE, Bodhidharma, a monk from India, went on a mission to China so he could spread the word about the virtues of meditation. During his demonstration at a temple, the eager monk shut his eyes, and several years later he awoke. Upset that he was feeling sleepy, he seized tea leaves from a tea bush and was awakened (pun intended) by its miraculous healing powers of feeling alert and focused. (There are different versions of this story, and it is unknown if he drank the tea or consumed tea leaves.) As the legend goes, the monk believed the tea allowed him to meditate without distraction and put him in a Zen-like state.[2]

In the 1600s, as tea authorities share, people of Europe were introduced to the tea of Asia. Initially, a tax on tea was pricey—and the beverage was appreciated by the wealthy. In time, demand for the drink with healing powers soared and tea was no longer just for the well-to-do—and it was enjoyed by more people. Coffeehouses were "in" and as the demand for tea soared, afternoon teas were "in" and not just for the elite.[3]

During the 1700s, as people in the tea industry around the world know and will gladly tell you, tea was noteworthy to English colonists, and the popularity of the drink continued to grow. Due to the desire for tea in America, England's high taxes soared for the commodity, causing an uproar among the Northeastern folks. The end result: an epic revolt—in an attempt to make tea accessible to everyone, rich or poor.[4]

The Boston Party Makes Its Move

As the story goes, one wintery evening in 1773, men dressed as Native Americans snuck onto British ships in the Boston Harbor. Without hesitation they tossed more than 300 chests of tea into the Atlantic Ocean. While not the only time tea was thrown overboard in protest of the British tax on tea, this event was so notable it was called the Boston Tea Party—and led to the Revolutionary War.

In the 1800s, American merchants grew aware of the vast demand for tea and the need to get it delivered quickly—consumers wanted it fresh and fast (not unlike the 21st century). Enter the time for ships called the "clippers"—boats capable of making a trip from Asia to the East Coast of the United States within months. This, in turn, made tea more readily available for tea drinkers.

THE ROOTS OF THE TEA PLANT

Welcome to Garden to Teacup 101—these facts are well-known to people behind tea, including growers and sellers. Tea does not grow on trees just anywhere. Tea is grown on tea estates or in tea gardens. Tea plants thrive in tropical and semitropical climates, where it will grow anywhere from sea level to 8,000 feet. It is a strong plant that'll grow in a variety of soil types. The best teas grow at a cooler, higher altitude and growers reap the reward.

Enter the tea tree, an evergreen from the *Camellia* family. Amazingly, tea bushes can grow up to a towering 50 feet, but are kept at a low and easy-to-tend-to three feet. The lifespan of a healthy tea tree is for more than a century. While there are at least 3,000 varieties of teas, like varieties of chocolate and coffee, their names are from where they are grown—like Ceylon or Assam black teas—around the world.

Greet "pluckers" . . . These are people, often locals, who remove by hand the top two leaves and leaf bud—a fine art that will lead to producing a fine tea. The tea plant grows new leaves, monikered a "flush," every one to two weeks. The end result: It will yield one pound of tea. (Note: A tea flush refers to tea growing seasons; first and second flushes are earlier in the season and preferred, as they are the highest quality.)

To make black tea, the leaves are withered and dried by air. Then, the juices are released by mechanical crushing methods, and then allowed to oxidize. As the oxygen is absorbed, the leaves turn from green to a darker color. The high-temperature drying causes the leaves to turn black. Oolong tea goes through the same process as black tea, except the leaves are not fermented all the way. Green tea is produced by steaming the leaves right away after plucking, and white tea is the least fermented.

After processing, tea—all types—is sorted into leaf grades. Samples are sent to tea buyers who purchase it through different means, including from the estates (perhaps this is why owners of tea companies are well traveled with tea tales to share). Once teas enter the United States, it is held in bonded warehouses until a tea examiner from the Food and Drug Administration gives the tea a thumbs-up. The teas are blended by tea manufacturers and packaged for sale.

In the 1900s, tea time hit America (as one who grew up in that century knows and experienced). On the East Coast, West Coast, in the South, and the Midwest, tea and tisanes continued to become a growing phenomenon for enjoyment, comfort, energy, health, and wellness.

Tea was and still is a mainstay around the globe—one of nature's special remedies. In the mid-20th century tea was found in specialty shops, health food stores, and Asian markets.

THE TEA ENTHUSIAST'S LEXICON

As you continue on your journey with me through the land of tea, these terms will be good to know as you are introduced to different teas.

Caffeine	The chemical in tea that creates a stimulating effect in the human brain and nervous system
Decaffeinated	Teas that do not contain caffeine (but not all caffeine can be eliminated)
Dessert tea	Uncommon flavors blended with sweet flavors (black tea with chocolate, caramel; chocolate rooibos)
Estate tea	A single-origin tea from a single geographical region; often bearing the name of origin (i.e., Assam, Ceylon)
Tisanes	Herbal or non-teas because they are derived from flowers, leaves, and barks of plants other than the tea plant
Whole-leaf teas	Teas that consist of leaves that are big and whole, unbroken

The Accidental Inventor(s) of the Tea Bag

As the popular story is told, Thomas Sullivan is the marketer behind the tea bag. In 1908, the New York marketer was on the quest for a more cost-effective way of distributing tea. Instead of the tins he tried putting samples in silk tea bags. Tea drinkers thought the tea bags were supposed to be used just like the metal infusers, by putting the bag into the pot—not dunked and tossed. Oops. It was a fateful event or "accident" and the convenient tea bag was created. But that's not the end of the tea bag birth . . .

According to some tea authorities, the tea bag may actually have been created by two women: Roberta C. Lawson and Mary Molaren of Wisconsin. Seven years prior to Mr. Sullivan's discovery, the duo filed a patent for a "Tea Leaf Holder" like a tea bag.[5]

Iced tea, America's favorite way of enjoying tea for more than a century, made its debut in 1904. It is no surprise that it was created in the hot summertime. As the story goes, the cold tea was created at the World's Fair in St. Louis. A merchant tried to make a profit from his hot tea but it was not selling. An attempt to pour the hot tea over ice attracted people because iced tea is refreshing and it was a novelty.

Nowadays, in the 21st century tea can be found not only in specialty shops, health food stores, and Asian markets, but also in mainstream grocery stores. Tea and tisanes have their own aisle, wellness teas are found in the health products aisle, and tea-infused products, including baked goods, beauty items, and cleaning products, are everywhere throughout stores.

Major producers of tea, including China, Japan, Sri Lanka, South America, and India, export their tea and tisanes to companies around the globe and in America. These days, much like yesteryear, tea's healing powers and potential as a versatile superfood render it in demand by people in the tea industry and consumers around the world.

OTHER PAST MEDICAL USES OF TEA

The use of tea from ancient times forward is backed up by the consensus of tea proponents. (If you're interested in more historical highlights, refer to the bibliography at the end of this book.)

Historical Users	Method/Tea	Uses
Sumerians[6]	Documented medicinal properties of plants	To treat different health ailments
Chinese	Drank green tea leaves	Health benefits
Chinese and Japanese monks	Drank tea	To stay alert
Chinese Ming Dynasty	Drank black and green teas	A lifestyle for pleasure
Chinese, Dutch	Tea	To treat headaches; alertness
People worldwide	All tea types	As a remedy for heart disease, immune system, nerves; enhance lifespan

OTHER TEA MILESTONES

Numerous books document that tea authorities and historians agree on the same time frames for when tea made its mark around the world. Here are a few highlights of when and how the healing powers of tea played a role in peoples' lives.

Year	What Happened	What It Did
221 C.E.–1911 C.E.	Chinese tea dynasties[7]	Usage of tea and its health virtues were shared by dynasties through centuries

400–600 A.D.	Chinese experiment with tea; adds spice to drinks	Shows people that tea has healing benefits
618–907	T'ang dynasty touts tea and it grows in popularity.	Tea begins to be used for its strong medicinal benefits
760–780	Lu Yu writes *The Classic of Tea.*	This book touts healing powers of tea.
1101–1125	Hui Tsung, Chinese emperor, becomes a tea advocate.	He writes about tea uses.
1518–1593	Physician and author pens book on healing powers of tea.	Shows how tea staves off anxiety, fights fat, and enhances mental focus
1600s	European settlers introduce tea to New England.	Tea is enjoyed in Asia and England for its relaxation and medicinal purposes
1657	Englishman Thomas Garway debuts his vision of tea and its health benefits in a in a poster ad.	The health merits of tea are circulated through England
1876	Thomas Lipton opens first shop in Glasgow, Scotland.	Paves the way for more coffeehouses and tea shops

These unforgettable milestones are inspiration for carrying on the tradition of tea and sharing its virtues with you. On a quest for an all-natural and simple iced tea creation, I used my own recipe, the one I've enjoyed throughout the years and back to the 20th century. This is a black tea (no bells and whistles) but I gave it a down-to-earth 21st-century healthy twist by adding honey, citrus, and mint. It's an easy-to-brew tea and one that will please your palate for four seasons, especially during the warm days of spring and summer.

Iced Tea with Citrus and Mint

This recipe is California-inspired from when I was in my twenties and lived in Fresno, a farming region in the central state where orange groves are plentiful. During the hot summer afternoons I'd drink iced orange pekoe (pronounced PECK-oh)—a grade of orthodox black tea—to get energized so I could enjoy riding a ten-speed bicycle accompanied by my soulmate with paws, a young and healthy black Labrador retriever, Stone Fox, who had dark brown soulful eyes and a smile to melt your heart. He'd run free through orange groves, and we'd race until we were whooped. From my backpack, I'd treat myself to cold tea in a plastic container and let my dog drink water from a hose or fountain outdoors to refresh ourselves.

4 cups water (fresh tap or filtered)
5 tea bags, orange pekoe (Harney & Sons—a blend of
Assam and Ceylon)
Granulated white sugar or honey to taste
Lemon or orange slices
Fresh mint

Bring 2 cups water to a boil and pour it over tea bags. Cover and brew 3 to 5 minutes. Remove tea bags and add 2 cups cold water. Stir. Pour into chilled, ice-filled tea mugs or glasses. Add sugar or honey to taste. Garnish with lemon slices and mint. Serves 4.

Going back to basic tea beverages sometimes is like embracing tradition that gets better with time. In the next chapter, "A Historical Testimony," I'll show you exactly how tea continues to get praise and why it's good enough to stock your pantry with for "... the best of times ... the worst of times," in the words of Charles Dickens's *A Tale of Two Cities.* You'll see why so many authors, including this one, turn to tea for inspiration and to find their Zen.

TEA-CENTRIC HEALING HINTS TO STEEP

✓ Tea's roots can be traced back centuries to Asia, including Japan and China, where tea leaves were brewed for their versatile virtues, from enhancing alertness to pleasure and medicinal remedies. . . .

✓ Tea was touted by Asian dynasties (more than 20) for its amazing healing powers, which eventually were recognized in other countries.

✓ By the 17th century, tea was praised in London by Europeans (especially royalty), who used tea for both relaxation and medicinal purposes.

✓ In the 18th century, tea made a big splash in America and continued to appeal to all regions around the country. The multipurpose tea plant was used to heal the mind, body, and spirit.

✓ The 19th and 20th centuries saw people from all countries embracing tea as a beverage—and preparing it differently in different cultures.

✓ Today, in the 21st century, tea is a superfood used as a beverage as well as infused in cuisine, beauty and cleaning products, and as home cures by people around the world.

PART 2

BLACK TEA

A Historical Testimony

Tea, though ridiculed by those who are naturally
coarse in their nervous sensibilities, will always be
the favorite beverage of the intellectual.
—Thomas de Quincey, *Confessions of an English Opium-Eater*

As a curious tween, I was introduced to black tea during school spring break. My friend's mother drove us to the Santa Cruz beach on Wednesdays because that was her day off. She was an okay lady, but I didn't like to eat her nondescript sandwiches served on sand. In hindsight I'd prefer sweet tea with fresh scones and jam and to be treated like a princess at the Ritz. Instead, I shared a pitcher of black tea (the plain dark stuff grown-ups drank). I plugged my nose and took a sip. I didn't love it, but I didn't hate it. It was bittersweet. Mrs. Cates said, "I put sugar in it." I nodded with approval. The brew made me feel like a teenager, so I indulged and pretended it was a fancier teacup. My hair frizzed from the steam of the tea (like it did when I encountered fog by the sea) while I waited for the liquid to cool, but I didn't care that day. Enjoying the novelty of the beverage made me feel noble and secure.

The tea (maybe it was both the sugar *and* caffeine) gave me a boost of confidence. I asked my friend if she wanted to rent a surfboard and try to ride the three-foot waves. We did it. That day was the beginning of my coming out of my shell and trying new things. Decades later, when I reminisce about trying to catch a wave, I give credit to the healing powers of tea—it gave me the nudge I needed to get physical for my personal well-being and sense of self.

During the sixties and seventies, black tea—which I learned to love—was popular. I drank it to get invigorated while traveling; and tea vendors in America were also explorers in the 20th-century tea industry. Pioneers in the world of teas understood the tea plant and its gifts to mankind. They knew that tea is versatile and healthful—both inside and outside the body. And these findings have been embraced and are now becoming the latest buzz to the mainstream audience.

In the 21st century, decades later, when I was a visitor at The Canadian Coffee & Tea Show in Vancouver, British Columbia, I attended classes on tea topics (such as "Comparative Tea Tasting" and "Trends and Opportunities in Sustainable Tea"). When we were discussing eco-friendly teas, I was unaware at the time of how progressive Lipton Tea (the tea I grew up on) had become (owned by Unilever and staying on top of its game offering earth-friendly tea[s]). And I, too, have continued to blossom in the land of tea.

TWO MEN IN A TEA INDUSTRY

The Man Behind Lipton Tea . . . The founder of this tea was named Thomas Lipton, aka "Sir Tea." The brand, now a staple in the United States, started in 1915 as Thomas J. Lipton, Inc. As I noted earlier, Lipton was the first tea box I saw as a child and the first tea type I drank.

As history tells it, the man behind Lipton Tea was born in Glasgow back in 1850. As a hard worker with a gift for sales, by his early twenties he had fine-tuned his business savvy and opened nearly two dozen shops. Tea was the product that helped him to gain his notoriety. Getting rid of the middleman, Sir Tea sold his own blend of tea in different amounts—and his tea was a grand success. Once Lipton's tea arrived abroad in the United States in the early 1900s, Lipton grew in epic proportions throughout the years into the 21st century.

A Lipton Tea researcher: Enter Peter Goggi. He began his career at Lipton Tea Company as a research chemist working on tea leaf, instant tea, and decaffeinated tea processes. In doing his work, he had his "experiments" evaluated by the Tea Tasters in Royal Estates Tea Company, the tea buying and blending division of Lipton. "It was there that I first observed tea tasting. I was not really cut out for bench-top research, so I had actually accepted a position at NYU as a graduate assistant in their Ph.D. program. Before I let Lipton know, the president of Royal Estates asked if I was interested in training to be a tea taster." The twist of fate involved working in Royal Estates and then living overseas training in the full tea supply chain. He happily accepted and lived in the U.K., Sri Lanka, and Kenya, with short stints in Malawi, India, and Indonesia.

In 2011, Peter retired from Unilever. As president of the Tea Association in 2016, Peter supports driving the tea and health message of the Tea Council to executing the growth agenda for the Specialty Tea Institute. As he does his work in the tea industry, the tea industry continues its work. . . .

TOP BRANDS PAVING THE TEA ROAD

I find it intriguing that some tea companies (and the people behind them) are pioneers in the tea industry since they are family-run and have ties back to the early 1800s or 1900s. Here, take a glance at some of my favorite commercial brands from A to Z:

Bigelow: Let me introduce you to Bigelow Tea Company, a family-owned business with roots in America—and a plantation in South Carolina. Their collection includes the popular category of teas, including black and green, as well as herbal teas, too. Tea bags in boxes of this brand are easily found at supermarkets. Also, the term "Healthy Antioxidants" is printed on the tea boxes that sit in my tea cupboard. I have a lot of boxes of this brand, including chamomile and salted black caramel.

Celestial Seasonings: Like Bigelow, this popular commercial tea brand is a household name in America. The tea company, which was established in 1969 in Colorado, uses herbs handpicked from the Rocky Mountains. It is known for their herbal tea collection but includes black, white, and green teas, too. Also, Celestial Seasonings has a wellness teas line and dozens of herbal teas that are available in supermarkets like Bigelow teas.

Harney & Sons: Another American family-owned tea company is this one, which goes back decades to 1983. Their packaging and presentation is very impressive for the consumer—and awards have been achieved for best tea company. A wide selection of teas and tisanes in tin cans will impress you as they do me; and they offer loose leaf, bags, and sachets. The tea is unforgettable because the blends are flavorful and aroma amazing—it's as good as it gets for tea lovers. What's more, tea masters will tell you Harney & Sons is a big name in the commercial tea bag industry *and* they stand out in the restaurant and hotel industry.

Tazo: This brand was once based in Portland, Oregon, but was picked up by Starbucks and is now not only well-known in the Pacific Northwest but around the world. En route to The Canadian Coffee & Tea Show, this was the brand of tea bags served to me in restaurants and hotels in Seattle, Washington. It is also available in my friendly Safeway grocery store.

Twinings: Much like the genesis of Lipton, this brand is linked to one man, Thomas Twining from London, and goes back to the early 1700s—and then branched out to being a major manufacturer of tea in the world. When I was tearoom hopping in Vancouver, British Columbia, a hot spot named The Urban Tea Merchant served Twinings tea. Ignorant of the man behind the tea brand, I asked for an interview . . . a few centuries too late. My face still turns red when I think about how the tea master must have been stunned by my tea history naïveté.

Some top commercial brands include Adagio and Tea Source. It's likely you're loyal to specific name brands, but it's never too late to broaden your tea repertoire and include specialty tea brands like Aiya America and Glenburn Tea District.

Dozens of smaller private-brand tea companies may please you, as will embracing household tea trademarks like the global commercial brand Lipton, which keeps up with consumer demands for tea varieties and earth-friendly tea products. Go ahead—go out of your comfort zone and be adventurous when in the land of tea.

TEA TIME WITH A TEA EDUCATOR EXTRAORDINAIRE

James Norwood Pratt is a celebrated tea authority. I had the pleasure to ask the go-to connoisseur questions about tea, past and present. As the author of *The Ultimate Tea Lover's Treasury*, it seemed apropos to engage in an exclusive interview with the man of books on tea love. He had me at the sentence: "There's nothing better for the human body than tea, but I feel its most valuable role is in promoting MENTAL health." Here, take a tea break and read about the tea master.

Q: *How and when did you fall into the world of tea?*
A: For Southerners, iced tea is an important food group. I've never been without it in one or another form. I started taking it seriously after publishing books on wine. Took to it in defense of my sobriety.

Q: *Do you live in San Francisco? Also, what role does tea play in your life right now, personally and professionally?*
A: I've been a San Franciscan since 1965. I greet the day with tea and consume it most waking hours—with friends or alone with Valerie, my wife. I've made my pleasure into my profession.

Q: *Black or white tea? Tell me why you feel they may be getting more attention in the 21st century versus green tea?*
A: White tea has only been discovered here in the past 20 years, the same period that's seen green tea sales soar. Black tea sales are also soaring, though it's the type with which we've long been most familiar. We're learning to love oolong and Pu-erh also.

Q: *You were named Honorary Director of the Imperial Tea Court, a Chinese teahouse founded in 1993 by Roy Fong in San Francisco, now located in the San Francisco Ferry Building. Please explain what this is exactly.*
A: Roy Fong is my teacher in China tea and I am his first—thus senior—student. Because of my enthusiasm over these newly available teas, Roy considered me the apostle of China tea to the "round-eyes." I've done my best to spread the word.

Q: What do you foresee happening in the tea industry within 10 years, 20 years?

A: America's tea renaissance since the 1990s has a long way to go before we can be called a tea-consuming society—but we're rapidly getting there.

Q: It's morning. Coffee or tea? Why?

A: Black tea from Yunnan starts my days—coffee ceased to be my friend in my fifties. Never swore it off—it just abandoned me.

Q: Is this your quote—exactly? "Taking tea is a moment of windless calm amid the bluster of daily events and has always been one of humanity's favorite pleasures. But beyond pleasure, tea can also provide glimpses of the ultimate reality, usually when we least expect any."

A: Yes, I wrote that. Tea is quiet and creates a quietness inside us when we drink it. To enter that quiet deeply is to meet oneself.

OTHER 20TH-TO-21ST-CENTURY MOVERS AND SHAKERS IN THE TEA AND HEALTH INDUSTRY

It is no surprise that in the 20th century to the present day, many people, not unlike Pratt, are behind the tea industry and making milestones as tea sweeps the world with its healing gifts from the tea plant.

Time Frame	What Did They Bring to the Tea Table?	Author/Doctor/ Researcher
20th–21st	He was the first true campaigner of tea, supporting the goodness of tea and its positive contribution to human health.	John Weisburger, MD, Ph.D.
20th–21st	Past president of the Southern Tea Company, co-chair of the Tea Association's Tea and Health Committee, one of America's foremost tea	Marty Kushner

experts on attention, work
performance, and creativity
with more than 55 years of
experience in the tea industry

Over 15 years	Bone loss and tea, research on bone diseases via complementary medicine, and alternative medicine, such as green tea	Chwan-Li Shen, Ph.D.
Since 1991	She has assisted the tea industry in creating awareness of the health benefits of tea; the industry attributes growth in both the green and black tea markets to her campaigns.	Louise Pollock, President, Pollock Communications
20th–21st	Scientist at Tufts University, research efforts focused on antioxidant nutrients and their dietary requirements in health promotion and disease prevention during the aging process. In 2012, he chaired the Fifth International Scientific Symposium on Tea & Human Health.	Jeffrey Blumberg, Ph.D.
Since 1991	Past president of the Tea Association of the U.S.A., Inc., driving force behind the International Symposia on Tea & Human Health	Joe Simrany
Since 2007	Cognitive benefits of tea, involved in several studies investigating the effects of tea ingredients	Suzanne Einother, Ph.D.

(*Source:* Peter F. Goggi, president, Tea Association of the U.S.A., Inc.)

Citrus-Spiked Black Tea

Black tea hot or cold is not only healthful, bold, and flavorful, but spiked with citrus it can be even more appealing, calming, and energizing any season of the year. Using a plain Lipton tea bag or a specialty black tea sachet or loose leaf tea is your choice but all forms can warm you up or cool you down and take you to that place where you can sit back and exhale.

1 cup water
1 tea bag, sachet, or 1 tablespoon loose leaf black tea
½ teaspoon lemon peel
½ teaspoon lime peel

Bring water to boil. Remove from heat. Add tea, citrus, and cover. Let steep for 3 to 5 minutes. Strain leaves and citrus peel. Serves one.

Now that I've put tea, nature's versatile superfood, on the table, it's time to take a closer look at its healthful ingredients like a sea diver (looking for hidden treasure) in the deep ocean. (As a good swimmer, I still skipped traveling over large bodies of water to Japan or China, but others do the work so I can share their findings.) So, what exactly makes black tea a superfood? I tackle this nutrition topic in the next chapter.

TEA-CENTRIC HEALING HINTS TO STEEP

✓ Different countries—not the United States—are known for their tea production because they contain the required environment. However, tea companies in America do sell source teas from around the world to all people, including health-conscious nuts and foodies.

✓ Classic tea companies, including Lipton and Bigelow, are holding their place in the progressive global tea industry.

✓ Tea producers are touted for their specialty teas, but in the present day they are also praised for sustainable tea and striving for a good work ethic for their workers in a growing earth-friendly industry.

✓ Medical doctors, scientists, and tea producers and companies, like health-conscious consumers (of all ages), are aware of the growing trend of tea.

✓ The tea industry in the 21st century has captured a worldwide audience and is touted for its healing powers. Still, more hard-hitting research is needed to convince the medical community about tea and its definitive usage for guarding against diseases.

Noteworthy Nutrients

*My hour for tea is half-past five, and my buttered
toast waits for nobody.*
—Wilkie Collins, *The Woman in White*

In the summers of the carefree sixties, during my early teenage years,
I'd spend time at my best friend's house around the corner. She lived
in a different world. Her backyard was an Adam and Eve picturesque
utopia, surrounded by fruit trees, flowers, an herbal garden, and a natural environment—not landscaped, no manicured lawn. I remember
my gal pal was often clad in overalls and barefoot, brewing tea in the
garden with her yellow dog, a Labrador mix off leash.

One morning when I paid Lois a visit she was brewing tea outside.
It wasn't the black stuff in the thermos I drank at the beach. The
black tea blend with a fruit tea made a bright orange-red-colored liquid inside a mason jar with a clamped lid, steeping in the sunshine.
She added light honey, slices of lemon, and ice cubes. The citrusy
aroma was welcoming and lingered in the air. She poured me a glass
mug of tea. With the morning sun, a Persian cat named Blue basking
on the porch, I felt a sense of calmness. She called it "Sun Tea" and it
enabled me to transcend to a peaceful place like sitting on a beach in
the sunshine, sipping tea in the Hawaiian Islands.

THEN AND NOW HISTORY OF BLACK TEA

If you're expecting a lot of history about the roots of black tea, you may be disappointed. While we know tea comes from the same plant—not a black tea plant—it's green tea in Asia that has been in the limelight since centuries ago. Black tea, though, was on hand in the Ming dynasty in the 16th century, most likely at a tea manufacturing plant in the Fujian Province. Black tea was circulating and gaining lots of followers in America during the early 19th century. And, of course, even I as a child recall black tea was served in households and restaurants throughout the United States during the 20th century.

These days, in the 21st century, black tea is still the number one favorite tea in America, as mentioned earlier. Americans drink more black tea—85 percent more than green tea, oolong, white and dark. Tea people tell me the most popular black teas include a breakfast tea (perhaps due to its energizing, feel-good caffeine), which includes English Breakfast, Irish Breakfast, and Earl Grey teas.

As I've noted in earlier chapters, black tea goes through the most processing. At a past Canadian Coffee & Tea Show in Vancouver, British Columbia, during one of the classes I attended we were offered a cupping time to taste different teas from different regions. It was the very first time I tasted black teas: Assam and Darjeeling—two black teas from provinces in India. If you desire to dig deeper there is a vast selection of specialty black teas to enjoy (similar to coffees or wines). Different black teas are limitless and include: Assam Organic, Steamed Darjeeling green tea, Ceylon Organic, and scented teas from China that use jasmine flowers or rose petals. But no matter where black tea comes from and how exotic it is, its compounds are what matters for health's sake.

Studies abound showing the nutrient benefits of black tea as we tea drinkers reap the healing powers, bold taste, and well-being of classic black tea—but that doesn't mean the black tea is full of nutrients visible to you when reading nutrition labels on a wide variety of tea boxes. Here's what you'll see if you do a search on the Internet and find what a cup of black, brewed tea contains:

Nutrition Facts:
Serving Size: 1 8-ounce cup (21 g)
Servings Per Container: 22

Amount per Serving:

Calories: 2

Total Fat: 0 g

Sodium: 0 mg

Total Carbohydrate: 0 g

Sugars: 0 g

Protein: 0 g

(*Source:* A variety of tea brands with nutrition labels on the box.)

When you look at a tea box to read the product nutrition label, often there is no nutrition label. The numbers are a dieter's fantasy: The tea contains almost no calories, no fat, no cholesterol, and no sodium. While it doesn't provide any good nutrients for you, the lack of calories, fat, sodium, and sugar is a good thing.

But the deal is, tea contains a lot more that is not listed on the label. Tea (all types) contain disease-fighting, anti-aging antioxidants, the good stuff found in nutrient-dense fresh fruits and vegetables, according to antioxidant researchers of stacks of tea, as well as health studies, medical doctors, and nutritionists who know tea is a super-food that can help keep heart disease, cancer, and obesity at bay. And it can do so much more.

During my tea research journey, I discovered some foods don't require nutrition labels, according to the FDA, and that can include tea. Many major tea brands do include nutrition facts and some feature "antioxidant" properties of tea. The complexity of tea and lack of nutritional data labels gets a bit more complex, so to speak. (For some health-related eco-friendly terms you'll see more and more on tea boxes, turn to chapter 17, "Teamania: Trends to Household Hints".)

"Black tea" or "green tea" may be all that is needed to read on a single-ingredient tea nutrition label as long as the only ingredient is *Camellia sinensis*. But beware, a box of herbal tea sometimes does not always provide every single ingredient. If you contact the manufacturer by phone or go online and do a search on a tea company's Web site and ask, for example, "Which herbal teas contain licorice root?" sometimes a list of the ingredients in their teas will pop up.

I love chamomile for its relaxing benefits, for instance, but one autumn afternoon I was blindsided by a new blend (Honey Vanilla Chamomile Herbal Tea) from a familiar brand I love. After one 12-ounce cup of the caffeine-free herbal tea, instead of feeling calm, my heart was racing—from a normal 60 beats per minute to 90 beats. I logged on to the company's Web site and read the variety of ingredients in the chamomile tea blend: licorice root was included. I recalled that this herb can cause hypertension for some people and it was obvious I am one of those people. So, I tossed the tea and now I only buy brands listing only "chamomile flowers," and I've continued my love affair with chamomile.

One dietitian I interviewed didn't have a whole lot of tea data to share, which brought me back to the days when I was writing about the health virtues of raw honey. This time around, I didn't want to debate, because there are studies, past and present, medical researchers at work as I write this book, and anecdotal evidence that goes back centuries pointing to the fact that tea does contain healing powers.

Tea is much more than a low-cal, refreshing glass of iced tea in the summertime and cup of hot black tea to warm up in the winter days. So, I chose to take her few words of wisdom and continue my trek in Tea World—a place where new findings happen constantly—showing us that the tea people of past centuries were onto something: The healing powers of tea do exist and the list of its benefits grows like tea plants. I went back to the tea masters who are aware of the healthful superfood. While reading the nutrition facts is similar to analyzing vinegars (not a lot to see on a nutrition label), these products do boast antioxidants and their properties do differ from tea to tisane and company to company—and the quality varies, too.

Remember, choose tea leaves and tea bags *before* instant tea powder and ready-to-drink teas (I can personally attest that these pre-bottled drinks that don't require brewing or preparation can be refreshing, flavorful, and energizing due to the sugar and caffeine). And note, with popular black tea, not unlike popular apple cider vinegar, the bigger the measurements the more nutrients you'll find.

More Tea, Please

Tea (black), brewed, prepared with tap water; 1 cup (8 fluid ounces) contains:

- 2.4 calories
- 0.7 from total carbohydrate
- 0.0 g from fat
- 0.0 from protein
- 0.7 from total carbohydrate
- 7.1 mg from total omega-3 fatty acids
- 2.4 mg from total omega-6 fatty acids
- 11.9 mcg from folate
- 0.9 mg from choline
- 7.1 mg from magnesium
- 2.4 mg from phosphorus
- 87.7 mg from potassium
- 7.1 mg from sodium
- 884 mcg from fluoride
- 236 g from water
- 47.4 from caffeine
- 4.7 from theobromine

Apparently, more tea equals more nutrients. One cup contains more good-for-you vitamins and minerals, water, and caffeine.

(*Source:* USDA SR-21 National Nutrient Database for Standard Reference)

So one cup of black tea—Americans still consume black tea more than all types of tea—may look like it isn't really that beneficial when it comes to the ingredients listed on a nutritional label. But if you include its antioxidants, then you've got something to write home about. Research on flavonoids lists tea as the top major food source of this key antioxidant among adults in the United States (from 1999–

2002 and 2007–2010). What's more, since green tea is not differenti-
ated from black tea in the research, all brewed tea was classified to be
black tea.[1]

DARK TEAS

Welcome to another complicated term in the land of teas. Tea masters introduced me to this type of tea—especially for the serious tea
drinker. Dark teas exclude black tea (oxidized not fermented) so it is
not a big category.

On a tea menu if it includes dark teas you may very well be greeted
by Pu-erh. The once banned Pu'erh tea (under the Tea Importation
Act of 1896) is finding its way into the American market. Though still
relatively unknown in the U.S., Pu'erh shows promise because of its
unique flavor and potential healing powers.

A favorite Tea Pu'er—for your gut—is popular amongst serious tea
drinkers and tea masters. Pu-erh or Pu'er, an aged tea commonly trans-
lated in the West as "black tea," is one that is favored amongst sophisticated tea proponents like Certified Tea Master Daniel Johnson,
L.Ac., based in Pittsburgh, Pennsylvania. His take on the dark loose
leaf fermented tea is in line with the literature about the dark tea. Its
healing benefits may help keep your cholesterol numbers and weight
in check—and it is a digestion aid. As the tea guru tells it, this tea is
grown from large leaf, ancient trees in Yunnan, China. "It contains
both pre- and probiotic qualities," he explains and notes it supports
our "digestive microbiome." Adds the tea master: Traditional Chinese
medicine touts its flavor to be warming, sweet, and slightly bitter.
"Being fermented," points out Johnson, "it is easy to absorb and digest." Not only does he find Pu'er represents the Earth element, he
also finds Pu'er grounding and balancing.

Refer to chapter 5, "Black Tea, You're Amazing!" to discover why
this tea type in different varieties is the beverage of choice for people
around the world, and not to ignore the age groups including millennials and baby boomers, who want to stay heart-healthy, lean, and live
longer, higher-quality lives.

Sun Tea

An easy way to brew tea from nature's gift is to use the sun for its heat—and brew tea naturally! This is my own spin-off recipe from the 20th century with an updated twist of citrus and honey—rich in immune-boosting vitamin C and antioxidants, a sweet donation from the honeybee.

6 cups cold water, fresh tap or spring
3 black tea bags (classic black or orange pekoe)
Glass container or jar (large enough to hold 48 ounces)
1 fruit tea bag (berry)
1¼ cups ice, small cubes
Orange wedges, for garnish
Mint leaves
6 8-ounce iced tea glasses
Orange blossom honey, to taste

   Place water and tea bags in a glass container or jar with a clamp lid, cover, and put in direct sunlight for three to five hours. Once sun brewed, remove the tea bags and chill tea in the refrigerator. Put ice cubes about one-fourth full into tea glasses. Pour tea over the ice and add orange wedges and mint leaves. Add honey. Serves six. (You can use Italian storage jars purchased online or in specialty stores.) Pair with scones or tea cookies. (Health Check: Nutritionists advise placing sun-brewed tea in the refrigerator, and tossing leftovers after 24 hours for safety's sake. Sun tea can end up full of bacteria—something you do not want to consume.)

   So, the question is: How does black tea, an ancient essential elixir that is available to us today, help your body inside and outside to prevent disease? Scientists, medical doctors, researchers, and tea masters share everything you want to know about this tea—from basic to specialty—and you'll find some sobering secrets in the next chapter.

TEA-CENTRIC HEALING HINTS TO STEEP

✓ In the 21st century, black tea, not unlike green tea, contains plenty of healthful antioxidants.

✓ Black tea does not contain a lot of vitamins and minerals, like herbal teas, but it is praised because it has no calories, no fat, no cholesterol, and no sodium.

✓ While more cause-and-effect medical research is needed to prove black tea is a definitive nutritional wonder, medical researchers, tea masters, and holistic doctors in the United States and around the world agree that there are some potential health virtues of black tea.

✓ The quality of black tea—its source and form (loose leaf or bags are advised)—is important in getting the most antioxidants.

✓ The total ingredients of quality tea paired with nutrient-rich clean foods (like in the Mediterranean diet) may help lower the risk of developing heart disease, diabetes, and cancer.

✓ Black tea is used for home cures, both drinking it and applying it topically. (See chapter 15 for more invaluable healing powers for your mind and body.)

Black Tea, You're Amazing!

Tea is one of the mainstays of civilization in this country.
  —George Orwell, *Smothered Under Journalism: 1946*

Though my first encounter with sun tea was sweet, drinking a cup of plain, strong black tea is an acquired taste. During the sixties, being Twiggy-thin was fashionable and young women, like me, were targets to follow the trend—and that included adding black tea to fad weight-loss diets. When I was 13, one Wednesday night my parents returned from the weekly grocery shopping and filled the fridge, freezer, and cupboards. I grabbed a handful of Oreo cookies and skipped to my bedroom, my special sanctuary I used to share with my older sister. As I twisted the chocolate cookies apart, then licked the filling off, she sipped black tea. Images of me as a plump tween haunted me: I wore a pink two-piece bathing suit with my rounded belly; my sibling rival sported a navy blue one-piece suit and a flat stomach. It was time to turn to a dieter's best friend—tea.

The next day after school, I went home and to the kitchen. I poured tap water into the stainless steel tea kettle and waited for the whistle. I took out one tea bag from the red-and-yellow Lipton box, and brewed my first cup of tea. When I took the first small sip of black liquid, it tasted bold and I scrunched my nose. The second sip was doable. I thought: "This stuff will help me get skinny." Sip by sip, afternoon by afternoon, I drank the hot brew. It foreshadowed my 1970s granola and tofu regime. I was moving on into the health food movement that led me into a world of becoming a vegetarian and teetotaler when I hitched and hiked around America.

And while I didn't know it then, later as a health author I discovered how and why tea—all types—can help keep weight in check. I was unwittingly consuming a beverage that was touted, past and present, for its plethora of health perks—not just a quick fix to fit into a miniskirt.

Black tea—the most popular tea in America—is touted for its heart-healthy benefits not unlike green tea—a potential cancer fighter. Dr. Joe Vinson told me that back in 1995, his first work on tea was directing graduate student research and he discovered that green tea compounds were the most powerful polyphenol antioxidants in a test tube model of heart disease. But black tea came into play when they conducted research for atherosclerosis (the buildup of fats on your artery walls, which can up your risk of artery disease and stroke)—and it was discovered both green tea *and* black tea were equally beneficial.

TEA AND THE BIG C

According to scientific research, cancer-fighting antioxidants that are found in both green tea and black tea may help lower the risk of developing cancers. Still, there is no definitive study that shows tea will prevent cancer at the present time, despite it showing promise as an anti-cancer superfood. So, it's the combination of an antioxidant-rich diet with fresh vegetables and fruits, and a healthy lifestyle (both genes and luck) that may also keep cancer at bay. Tea is not a single magic bullet or a cancer cure.

How It Works: Still, past and ongoing research is in the works to find out if drinking black tea is helping humans lower the risk of developing cancer. More than 3,000 published research studies exist that evaluate the role tea and health-promoting compounds, such as epigallocatechin gallate (EGCG), also known as epigallocatechin-3 gallate (a type of catechin mentioned earlier), may play in cancers of various types.[1]

One study found that women who consumed the equivalent of 2.5 cups of tea per day had a 60 percent reduction in rectal cancer risk, compared with women who drank fewer than 1.2 cups of tea daily.

Research continues to confirm that black tea may lower the risk of this cancer.[2]

Ongoing scientific studies and published articles are linked to the infection-fighting properties of tea. And the compound from tea—EGCG—is touted for inhibiting the growth of tumor cells.

What You Can Do: Neither one nor a dozen cups of black tea per day is a cure-all for keeping cancer at bay for a lifetime—but it can't hurt to incorporate it into your diet. The National Cancer Institute and American Cancer Society are aware of tea and cancer-fighting potential but they do not endorse it as miracle cure. But, eating 4½ cups of fruits and vegetables per day (recommended by the American Cancer Society) may help you guard against cancer.

And black tea—the loose leaf or bags—brewed—paired with anti-cancer superfoods found in the Mediterranean diet together can be the beginning of an arsenal for you to keep the big "C" out of your life. And note, both organizations—the American Cancer Society and National Cancer Institute—are aware of the healing powers of green tea and its potential to help lower the risk of developing cancer, but they claim more research is needed.

TEA AND DIABETES

People who drink tea on a regular basis are believed to engage in a healthier lifestyle, good diet, and exercise, maintain a healthy weight—all factors that may help keep blood sugars regulated and keep type 2 diabetes at bay. It's not just tea that will prevent you from getting a diabetes diagnosis but it may be a superfood that can help keep diabetes out of your life.

How It Works: The Health Council of the Netherlands believes drinking three or four cups of tea (black or green) might boost your health by staving off diseases including diabetes. Evidently, drinking tea has a similar effect to eating antioxidant-rich fruits which can lower your blood pressure and help keep bad cholesterol from clogging your arteries.[3]

Past research published in the *British Medical Journal* shows that drinking black tea may lessen your odds of being a diabetes statistic. The researchers gleaned information from 50 countries and discovered black tea was linked to a lower risk of developing diabetes.[4]

What You Can Do: Drinking black tea may help keep type 2 diabetes at bay. Eating a healthy Mediterranean diet, getting regular exercise, and maintaining a healthy lifestyle and ideal weight can all help keep your blood sugar levels steady, too.

TEA AND HEART DISEASE

In stacks of studies, black tea is touted to help you lower the risk of developing heart disease. Researchers discovered drinking three or more cups of black tea per day have lowered the odds of developing heart disease or stroke.[5]

But the healing powers of black tea—*and* green, white, and oolong—are linked to cardiovascular health/disease overlap, points out Jeffrey Blumberg, Ph.D. "This is based on a substantial body of evidence, not just one recent study."

Still, black tea is touted for its promising heart-healthy benefits and continues to get kudos for its potential to aid in heart health, from helping blood vessels function, to preventing stroke and heart attack.[6]

How It Works: Drinking black tea on a regular basis may also lower the risk of developing bad cholesterol (the stuff that clogs your arteries, which can lead to heart attack) and high blood pressure, improve blood vessel function, reduce inflammation, and lessen the risk of blood clots. According to scientific research, cancer-fighting antioxidants that are found in black tea may help lower the risk of developing heart problems, too. It's the combination of heart-healthy antioxidants (theaflavins and thearubinins) in black tea and a healthy lifestyle that may protect you against heart disease—but studies do show drinking black tea on a regular basis is not to be ignored either.

Drinking tea can also reduce heart attack risk and lower low-density lipoprotein (LDL) "bad" cholesterol, with perks seen with just one cup up to six cups a day. One past study shows drinking black tea can lower risk of stroke in both women and men.[7]

What's more, a study published in the *American Journal of Clinical Nutrition* reveals that again black tea comes through and reduced blood pressure, and among hypertensive people it helped counteract the negative effects of a high-fat meal on blood pressure and arterial blood flow.[8]

What You Can Do: Since the jury is still out on the exact amount of black tea we're advised to drink each day—although some research points to three to five cups daily—moderation is the best recommendation among tea proponents and medical doctors (who advise widening your tea and tisanes regime), especially if you are caffeine-sensitive.

THE WORLD OF CHAI

During my journey at the Canadian Coffee & Tea Show, I stopped at a busy booth to receive a sample of chai. Prana Chai North America Managing Director Brian Haas offered me a cup of warm and delicious chai (also known as masala chai) made with soy milk that left me thinking: "More please." I was pleasantly surprised—but he was not. Once back home I interviewed the chai expert and discovered his link to this type of black tea goes back and faraway. Here, let me share his experience that led him fall into the world of chai. . . .

Brian traveled in India for three months, where he was first introduced to masala chai. "I grew to appreciate this style of tea and learned how to prepare it from several families I stayed with during that trip." Years later while living in New York, he was a frequent shopper at an Indian market in the East Village, where he could buy traditional ingredients and get tips on improving his masala chai recipe while perfecting both the brewing process and the beverage for years before coming into the chai industry.

The chai advocate is aware that tea, spices, and honey boast healing powers due to its myriad of nutrients—and he adds "many people find the combination of all to have a calming effect." Brian also points out, "People are also responding favorably to a more modest level of sweetness with no added sugars or artificial preservatives. Healthier alternatives are expanding the market for chai because those uninterested in the sugary options now have alternatives they can embrace." Also, he adds, "It's simply delicious. There's a reason it's been so popular in India and other countries for so long."

Brian notes soy, almond, and macadamia nut milks work well because they all have a taste and consistency that complement chai and accentuate the flavors from our tea (black Ceylon) and spices (cinnamon, cardamom, star anise, peppercorns, cloves, and fresh ginger). Not to forget honey, he adds, pointing out that each ingredient boasts medicinal properties that have long been used in Ayurvedic medicine and add to the many benefits that tea on its own already offers, and which he believes (I agree) taste amazing together.

Black Tea Types . . .

Assam: At the Canadian Coffee & Tea Show we tasted estate teas in the Comparative Tea Tasting class. We tasted Assam, Bukhial TGFOP (an acronym for Tippy Golden Flower Orange Pekoe, the main grade of Darjeeling and Assam.) A top Assam tea estate in India, it is bold, malty, and amazing for serious tea drinkers and tea lovers, like you and me. Assam tea is a popular black tea around the globe. It can enhance alertness due to its caffeine, which is helpful for both body and mind.

Ceylon: From Sri Lanka, this is an orange-colored cuppa. It has a flowery scent, and light aftertaste. Like black teas, this popular one can be used solo or in blends—which I have experienced in many flavored black teas that I prefer. It is heart-healthy due to its antioxidants.

Darjeeling: Found in the high Himalayas, this tea is amber-colored and has a fresh, clean taste (and I had the pleasure to taste it, too, at the Coffee & Tea Show. The Darjeeling Ambootia SFTGFOP (Special Finest Tippy Golden Flowery Orange Pekoe 1. Superlative grade.) was from India, like the Assam. It has the healing powers of other black teas but also enhances digestion.

Keemun: A quality black tea from China, and popular in the West, it is often used as a base in specialty black flavored teas. It's touted for its powers to aid in digestion but in a black flavored tea blend it has potential to deliver much more. Keemun is used for different blends, a light tea with floral and smoky notes.

FLAVORED (AND BLENDED) BLACK TEAS

Welcome to flavored teas, which in a nutshell mean any tea (not tisane) that has flavor added to it—the two most common types of teas in this category are black tea and green tea. Other flavored teas do exist in the tea market, such as white tea with berries, but they aren't as popular.

Tea master Daniel Johnson agrees with me and other tea proponents that flavored black teas are popular and will continue to attract consumers. The wide variety of these tasty teas can and are created to match the desired flavor profile of many new audiences, including baby boomers, like me, who for decades only drank basic black tea. In my pantry I have many flavored black teas—some from Harney & Sons. Paris, for one, is a fruity black tea with vanilla and caramel flavors. Valentine's Blend is a chocolate black tea with pink rosebuds and China black tea is the base.

Here is a short list of black flavored and scented teas that are often blended with other teas and tisanes for the fun and health of it.

Constant Comment: The familiar black-and-red box of tea bags welcomed me decades ago in kitchen cupboards of the well-to-do. The spicy black tea flavored with clove, cinnamon, and orange peel not only is pleasing to the palate (hot or iced) but it was my "constant" energizing helper during toilet-scrubbing college days. It is a popular flavored black tea in America and it did give me physical and mental stamina (especially when I had to pull an all-nighter writing features for the school newspaper).

Earl Grey: Back in the 1800s this tea was made with black teas, but now green, oolong, and even white are used also with oil such as bergamot. It's not uncommon for Earl Grey to also have sweet floral and citrus notes. This black flavored tea is commonly used in both cooking and baking.

English Breakfast: A brisk blend of Chinese Keemun and Yunnan blacks, Indian Ceylons. This tea, one that has been in my pantry more than once, is popular among Brits in England and throughout the United States. Like Assam, its caffeine is welcomed when a mental or physical boost is needed. It's a fine tea for any season, anytime when you want a familiar tea with a familiar taste you can count on for follow-through.

Irish Breakfast: This black tea, like English Breakfast, is also strong, a perfect brew for a hearty breakfast in the morning. As an Irish Catholic girl, I always make a pot of Irish Breakfast for Saint Patrick's Day *and* on crisp autumn mornings or cold winter days. It's a fine tea to give you a lift and pairs with pastries at afternoon tea. Like energizing black teas it boosts brainpower and physical energy—day or night.

Orange Pekoe: This known black tea, like Irish Breakfast, which I drank and liked in my lean years throughout my college days, undergraduate and graduate school, is orange in color and has a bold flavor. It is a perfect brew for much-needed alertness and a popular tea in America. As an adult this was one of my black teas of choice and readily available on the shelves at supermarkets, coffee shops, and in restaurants.

KOMBUCHA: A FERMENTED HEALTHY BLACK TEA

While black flavored and scented teas have a place in the land of teas, a special type of fermented black tea is gaining in popularity. Meet Hannah Crum, coauthor of *The Big Book of Kombucha: Brewing, Flavoring, and Enjoying the Health Benefits of Fermented Tea* (Storey Publishing, 2016). She is the kombucha pundit to dish on this fermented tea—considered a black tea like Pu'er—that is getting a lot of attention—and for good reason.

So, what *exactly* is kombucha tea, anyhow? "Kombucha is fermented tea—just like yogurt is fermented milk and sauerkraut is fermented cabbage," answers Crum, who explains it is fermented using a culture called a SCOBY (Symbiotic Culture of Bacteria and Yeast) that converts the tea and sugar into a beverage full of healthy acids and good microorganisms. The top healing powers of drinking kombucha may be better energy, better immunity, and just making you better. It's believed, says Crum, "the healthy acids, enzymes, and microdoses of bioavailable nutrition produced by the fermentation process support healthy liver function and provide nutrition in a living form," all linked to the promise of feeling better.

Kombucha tea, adds Crum, is mild tea "vinegar" and can have a tangy flavor that many find refreshing. She shares her loyalty to the tea: "I drink sixteen ounces of kombucha a day; my husband and partner drinks thirty-two ounces a day. Trust YOUR gut!" (See chapter 18 for cautions about this popular tea.)

Pot of Tea & Biscuits

❖ ❖ ❖

This quick-and-easy classic brew (a black tea blend that is common around the globe) paired with biscuits is perfect year-round. Here is an original recipe from my friend and mentor, an old-school Italian woman who bakes with olive oil. The original recipe calls for olive oil, but I include homemade honey butter for a sweet flavor and richness to savor.

4 cups water
4 tablespoons Earl Grey or Irish Breakfast Tea (loose leaf)
Lemon slices
Honey

In a tea kettle heat water until it comes to a full boil or kettle whistles. Remove from stovetop. Rinse teapot with hot water, and then pour tea kettle water into teapot. Place tea into strainer. Steep for 5 minutes and remove leaves. Pour into cups. Add lemon and honey. Serves 4.

Mini Buttermilk Biscuits

1 cup flour
1 teaspoon baking powder
½ teaspoon baking soda
½ teaspoon salt
3 tablespoons olive oil (Marsala or Sciabica)
¼ cup buttermilk

In a mixing bowl add dry ingredients (flour, baking powder, baking soda, and salt). Make a well in the center. Add olive oil and buttermilk. Stir until dough holds together. Turn dough onto a lightly floured surface, pat down to ½ inch thick. Cut out 12 biscuits with a 1-inch cutter; place on greased baking sheet. Bake in a 375-degree oven for 14 to 16 minutes or until golden. Serve warm. May be baked in a mini-muffin pan. Makes 12.

(*Courtesy*: Gemma Sanita Sciabica, *Cooking with California Olive Oil: Popular Recipes*)

For an extra touch to these biscuits with tea, I created my own recipe of Honey Butter (like I loved to eat on the warm golden corn bread at Marie Callender's Restaurant & Bakery).

Honey Butter: In a bowl mix ½ cup European sea salt butter with ¼ cup honey. Put into a small container with a lid and refrigerate. It pairs well with biscuits, corn bread, muffins, and scones.

In the next chapter, I'll show you how white tea—the "new" tea on the block—continues to get a thumbs-up in studies, by tea merchants, consumers—and me. It's the pureness that won my taste buds, heart, and soul—and may be one of your favorite types of tea, too. While black tea is familiar (and can be special) like fine coffee, imagine if you broaden your horizons and add different tea types, such as white tea—which does contain both medicinal properties and a lighter distinct flavor from black tea.

Take a look at Part 3, "White Tea," to see my refreshing findings of the world of white tea, and you can discover how you, too, can nourish your body, mind, and spirit without going to China to savor a rare specialty tea that deserves (and is getting) more recognition for its potential healing powers from head to toe (literally!).

TEA-CENTRIC HEALING HINTS TO STEEP

✓ Black tea may help lower the risk of developing cancers, reduce bad cholesterol, boost immunity, and much more.
✓ Black tea and its powers are acknowledged around the world as a healing medicine.
✓ Not unlike white and green tea, black tea heals in a variety of ways—thanks to its antioxidants, and other amazing properties.
✓ Despite its caffeine content black tea can calm your nerves due to its compound L-theanine.

BLACK TEA KEEPS THE DOCTOR AWAY

Disease	How Black Tea Works
Cancer	Phenols in black tea act as disease-fighting antioxidants to hinder the cancer process and may reduce certain cancers.
Diabetes	Black tea may cut the amount of "bad" LDL cholesterol in the blood, which may lower the risk of developing type 2 diabetes.
Heart Disease	Antioxidants in dark tea help to lower the risk of high blood pressure and high cholesterol.

PART 3

WHITE TEA

White Tea Revolution

*I believe it is customary in good society to
take some slight refreshment at five o'clock.*
—Oscar Wilde, *The Importance of Being Earnest*

Black tea did play a role in my diet repertoire during my mid-teenage years while growing up in "disturbia" (a place morphing into rules, sibling rivalry, and change). During the post-hippie sixties, at 17, I was looking for adventure outside of San Jose. Hitching and hiking to San Francisco, a place of diversity in people and cuisine, opened up a new world and a new tea for me.

One night I knocked on the door of a young couple; the two had invited me to be their renter when I decided to move out of my parents' home. I was welcomed by a friendly hippie-ish couple and entered their Victorian house in North Beach.

That evening in the city—no longer a suburbs girl—the man with a long ponytail, beard, and lanky body and his fiancée made me feel at home. The couple had leftover Chinese food from a new Asian restaurant in North Beach. Egg rolls and fried rice greeted me. We sat cross-legged on pillows laid out on the floor with a round table full of food and tea. We drank tea from a specialty shop in Chinatown, served from a ceramic pot. I was told it was a white tea (it was rare in the 1970s unless you had connections to royalty in China; so it is unknown if I was treated to the real stuff). It was mild and sweet, foreign to me—and from loose leaves, not a tea bag, served in mini white tea-cups without handles. After we ate, the woman took my cup, turned it over on a saucer and back upright. She read my tea leaves. After dinner, I left on my own to walk through the streets of the city. I was mesmerized by the glitter, strange faces, and the fast beat that wasn't part of suburban life. Riding trolley cars, talking to strangers, and sitting in a poetry reading were things I did and enjoyed. It was the energetic feeling, probably from the multiple cups of tea I drank, that made the nightlife vibrant and come alive.

Is White Tea the New Brew on the Block?

While black tea may be the most widely used tea in U.S. history, and green tea has been touted in past medical studies, white tea, its forgotten cousin, was used as well in past centuries, as discussed in the past chapters. White tea, also derived from *Camellia sinensis* (not a white plant as I imagined), attracts a select group of people. It's considered a rare tea—and is often used in blends of specialty teas. It may just be a late bloomer to blossom in the United States, as I see it—and if not—all the more for purists, like me (just kidding).

Finding its roots is not an easy task. I did make my research rounds to reference librarians, tea historians, and tea proponents, but the history of white tea is sketchy—whether you're talking decades ago or centuries ago. As the legend goes, youthful or magical and pure tea pickers plucked the tea plant buds, which led to selling tea touting its powers.[1]

Many theories of the outing of white tea vary. But piecing together tidbits of history (like rumors of something that is intriguing), we find the roots of white tea are from China. While there are more than 20 dynasties, some tea proponents believe the pure tea was available by the 12th century if not before. It was also believed white tea may have been royalty's favorite tea selection. It has been said by tea proponents that white tea may be linked later to the Qing dynasty in 1796. During this time, teas were produced from loose leaves and made from chaicha, a mixed-variety tea bush—and they were not processed like other China teas. As time passed, by the late 19th and early 20th centuries, white tea varieties such as silver needles and white peony were produced but still considered rare, veteran tea proponents will tell you.

In the late 19th century different types of white tea were created. One tea historian told me that white tea was not readily available in the 20th century in the United States. But in the 21st century, white tea is still considered rare, whether you notice the lack of it in Midwest America or in medical research. But its nutritional perks are of interest to both medicinal research and health-conscious people who are always on the quest for the superfood to love.

White tea definitely boasts disease-fighting antioxidants (as I'll show you in the next chapter) but my question is: Where are the human studies to prove its virtues? I love white tea—and it does have some wonderful benefits (as you'll see a bit later). So, I went to the tea wizard, Peter Goggi, president of the Tea Association of the U.S.A., and I asked for a prediction on white tea. "Will it ever get more kudos in medical research and more love from tea lovers?" And I waited for the answer.

"White tea, though popular," says Goggi, "is not consumed to a great extent as compared to green tea. Most research work surrounds green tea and black tea." He notes the big health virtues of these two popular teas which I note, too, but he points out the statistics stacked against the white stuff. "Black and green tea consumption comprises about ninety to ninety-five percent of the world's production/consumption, so while white tea is growing in popularity, its impact on human health would be minimal as total consumption is very low."

While sipping a fresh cup of Silver Needles in a white 16-ounce ceramic cup, which takes me back to a cozy birthday night with a pot of signature white tea at the Fairmont Hotel in Vancouver, British Columbia, I continue to digest Goggi's forecast for my favorite tea.

"White tea will continue to grow," he says, "but only in the specialty segment. It is very light and delicate in both appearance and flavor, but it will take some time for mainstream consumers to embrace this," he explains. "Further," adds Goggi, "the amount of white tea produced in the world is very small. Even in China, which makes up about ten percent of the world's tea, white tea represents less than one percent (.75 percent) of their production, meaning that it is less than .075 percent of the world's tea."

As I savor the mild flavor of my late-morning brew (made from loose leaf), and prepare to share my nutritional, health, home cures, beauty, and eco-friendly findings about my tea flavor of the century (another cup of white tea, please), tea savvy Goggi's words of wisdom remind me of a time when I wrote about specialty balsamic vinegar in *The Healing Powers of Vinegar* (not a lot of human studies, either). But the less popular specialty vinegar with anecdotal healing powers like red wine vinegar (after the publication of the first edition of my book in 2000) graced the cover and content of national magazines and Food Network chefs flaunt the rare vinegar in their dishes. So, while Goggi's words ring practical, I will remain idealistic and predict this ancient-day tea will become more in demand in the coming years, decades, and centuries. Here's why you may want this dream to come true.

A New Look at an Old Tea

We know white tea has Asian roots that go back centuries. Although black and white tea come from the same tea plant (*Camellia sinensis*), white tea is considered to be healthier and have its own healing powers, perhaps because it's the lesser processed tea since it comes from un-opened buds of tea shoots. I love that it is a much lighter beverage than bold black and dark teas, but note it's not white, it is a pale yellow color.

It's not rocket science to understand that since white tea is plucked earlier than black tea, it's less processed—and that means it is more pure, it contains more antioxidants. What's more, since it's antioxidant-rich it is a good tea to help maintain good health and lower the risk of developing cancer and heart disease—two culprits that affect people of all ages but increase as we age.

Speaking of age, I asked Goggi if back in the seventies and eighties it was possible to get white tea in health food stores or Chinatowns such as in San Francisco and New York City. His reply is similar to what tea historians and tea researchers told me. "Possibly, yes, but very unlikely," he says. "White tea was produced only in China, and tea from China wasn't allowed in the U.S. until circa 1974. At that time, the Chinese government was far more interested in finding markets for its major production volumes, green and black teas; white teas for export became available later in the 1990s."

In a tea bag, so to speak, we've come a long way when it comes to white tea and demand. Today, you can go to the supermarket and in the tea and coffee aisle you'll most likely find a few tea and/or tea blends with white tea. In the soap aisle you'll find dish soaps infused with white tea extract and the same for the beauty aisle with its beauty and bath products. And, keep in mind, "the night is young" (as the character pointed out in *Three Days of the Condor*)—which leads me to believe anything is possible, including an increase in demand of white tea.

WHITE TEA TYPES

At the Canadian Coffee & Tea Show, during the Comparative Tea Tasting session, I was served white tea (silver frost from the Emrock Estate in Kenya). It was smooth, sweet, light, and clean—and I wanted more, not just a small tasting cup portion. But there is white tea in my tea cupboard so I can drink up different varieties. Here, take a peek. . . .

Silver Needle: Another Chinese tea, this white tea is the most popular and well-respected white variety. It's called its name because of the needlelike look of the buds from a tea bush. Harvested in the early springtime, it is the most costly due to the fact that it may be the finest of white teas. Not to forget it's plentiful in disease-fighting antioxidants.

White Darjeeling: Like the popular Silver Needle that is in a tin container safe inside my tea cupboard, this tea was made in India. It contains more caffeine and fewer antioxidants—it's ideal if you want to get a physical and mental boost, but other white teas may be more healthful.

White Peony: This is a mild white tea. Its roots are from buds and two leaves. It contains nutty notes and makes a light-colored cup of tea. This type of white tea is often found in a fruit blend that is refreshing in the summertime or healing in the wintertime with its immune-boosting antioxidants.

In the next chapter, you'll come with me into the less chartered waters of white tea and its good-for-you ingredients, a place that is not as familiar as black tea to medical researchers, doctors, and people around the world, past and present. This tea type, however, is gaining popularity and has been studied but not a lot and not in big, hard-hitting research studies using humans. While the jury is still out on its health merits, findings in studies, folklore, and anecdotal evidence (not unlike ancient superfoods vinegar and honey) show promise. It has its place in my diet regime and it could for you, too.

White Tea Spring Rolls

This recipe is a little exotic and big on fun. Chinese take-out is nothing new but making Asian cuisine at home is newsworthy. True, it does take effort and more time than picking up spring rolls made for you, but if you do it yourself, there is a reward of controlling the ingredients—and adding fresh vegetables to white tea makes these babies delicious. Thanks to the tea master who provided this recipe, it's a keeper. Pair the spring rolls with a pot of green or oolong tea for a tasty snack, or include these rolls with other Asian foods for a meal.

2 tablespoons organic tea seed oil
1 tablespoon minced garlic
½ cup bean sprouts
½ tablespoon fresh ginger, grated
1 carrot, grated
2 cups shredded cabbage
2 ounces bean thread noodles, blanched and chopped
2 tablespoons hoisin sauce
1 tablespoon oyster sauce
*4 tablespoons finely chopped white tea (TCTC Bai Mu
    Dan, or loose, unflavored white tea)*
*Spring roll wrappers (found in refrigerator section of
    vegetable area in grocery store)*
1–2 tablespoons organic tea seed oil, for frying

Heat 2 tablespoons of oil in a skillet over high heat. Add the garlic, bean sprouts, ginger, carrot, and cabbage. Cook just until the cabbage is soft, 2–3 minutes. Add noodles. Stir in the hoisin and oyster sauces. Remove from heat and allow to cool. Toss in the chopped tea. Lay a spring roll wrapper on a flat surface on an angle so it looks like a diamond. Spoon 2 tablespoons of the filling near the bottom corner of the wrapper and fold up to cover the filling. Fold in the 2 sides and brush the top half with water and roll to form a tight cylinder. Pour enough tea seed oil to fill one inch of the skillet and heat to 350 degrees F. Fry the spring rolls for 2 minutes, turning to cook all sides. Drain on paper towels before serving. Makes 16 spring rolls. Serves 4.

(*Courtesy:* The Cozy Tea Cart)

TEA-CENTRIC HEALING HINTS TO STEEP

✓ White tea is one of the teas listed in tea types but it isn't as popular as black or green teas for different reasons, including price and limited production.

✓ The demand for white tea may expand around the world but it likely will remain in the demand of people who love specialty teas.

✓ Research studies on the healing powers of white tea have been limited, most likely due to its high price and low(er) consumption (like balsamic vinegar).

✓ While white tea is not the top tea on tea menus around the globe, anything is possible and the demand for it may grow in the future.

The Old and New
Incredible Ingredients

Tea should be taken in solitude.
—C. S. Lewis, *Surprised by Joy*

White tea, like I may have been gifted in San Francisco, was a refreshing beverage. I liked its natural sweetness, and subtle, savory flavor. The novelty of it made me feel like I traveled to China, no longer a just a Northern Californian–black-brew-with-sugar novice tea drinker. After days of living and loving The City, I journeyed south to Newport Beach, a warm beach town; and iced tea was a popular drink I sipped at a restaurant where I worked as a waitress. I met a piano player who was born and raised in Taiwan. He invited me to his apartment, where he made stir-fry vegetables and a pot of tea—"It's a blend of white tea and green tea," he told me. When I poured the light-colored liquid into my cup, I was inhibited by the unique tea. It overflowed out of the teacup and onto the table like the scene in the film *2012* when the elderly monk put too much tea into the boy's teacup—showing that he needed to keep an open mind—as I tried to do.

Intrigued with the blended tea, salty ocean air—lingering conversation—clean food with an Asian twist, I was in a happy place. I was enjoying a brew I never drank as a kid, tween, or teen—it was my new cup of tea. When I left that night, I was given the loose leaves in a packet, which I later found in my backpack.

WHITE TEA NUTRITION FACTS

If you take a look at a nutritional label on a box of white tea bags (not a tea blend), you will wonder why I give attention to this type of tea. It's no different from looking at a nutrition label on a box of black tea or green tea. It will tell you that it comes from the tea plant. Also, it does not contain added sugar or artificial colorings. Plus, it is organically grown. And, like black tea or green tea, if you look at the nutrition label on a white tea box, there will be an absence of ingredients such as vitamins and minerals per serving size. But that does not mean white tea is void of nutritional value.

Okay, okay, I know it will read zero for all the major nutrient groups listed on the label but wait, there's more. Think coffee and honey—both have a class act of antioxidants that show up in medical studies but not on a nutrition label of a bag of coffee beans or a jar of honey.

A NEW CLASS OF NUTRIENTS

So are you wondering where's the good stuff—the antioxidants? At the present time there isn't a chart like for black tea or green tea listing the ingredients of white tea. Nobody seems to provide an easy-to-decode chart of all the antioxidants in this rare brew from China. It seems the unanimous opinion is, according to medical doctors, researchers, and tea historians, green tea *and* less oxidized white tea contain more polyphenols than oolong and black tea.

I have also noticed a trend amongst tea proponents whom I have talked to and they tell me that the type of tea you drink isn't as crucial as the idea that you incorporate tea into your diet. Because the fact is *all* teas have many of the same healing powers.[1]

But I decided to dig deeper into the nutritional underground world of white tea and see if it contains more antioxidants than black tea, similar to the less used red wine vinegar versus the more popular apple cider vinegar. But even this popular vinegar, an ancient remedy that works wonders, boasts more folklore and anecdotal evidence for its health benefits than hard-hitting medical studies.

WELCOME TO WHITE TEA POLYPHENOLS

You'll find stacks of studies about the antioxidants of green and black teas on human health, but less is known about white tea, which is known as the rarest and the least processed. Researchers in Italy conducted a study published in *Food Chemistry* showing proof in how powerful white tea antioxidants (polyphenols) can be in white, green, and black tea—and the findings are surprising. The antioxidant epigallocatechin-3-gallate (EGCG) has been pinpointed as the major polyphenol player in *both* white and green teas. But there's more! Other disease-fighting antioxidants including catechins, EGCG, gallic acid, caffeine, and theobromine—which can do your body good from head to toe—were discovered to be present in higher levels in white tea than its counterparts black and green teas.[2]

FIVE QUESTIONS FOR
DR. JOE VINSON—AN ANTIOXIDANT WIZARD

Enter the good doctor. I had the chance to have a virtual cup of tea (he drank black tea flavored with caramel) and interview Joe A. Vinson, Ph.D., from the University of Scranton in Pennsylvania. Author and researcher of hundreds of studies about the healing powers of superfoods, he dishes on tea—including white tea—even though he fancies flavored black tea for taste, and drinks one 8-ounce cup of black or green tea each day. So, will white tea pass green and black teas and one day be the number one healing tea—or not? Read on to see what the antioxidant specialist brings to the tea table to me for you.

Q: *Which type of tea—black or white—is full of the most antioxidants? Why does black tea continue to get more press than white tea?*

A: White tea has slightly more antioxidants but the chemical nature of the antioxidants is quite different. White tea is chemically more similar to green tea than black tea. White tea has very few scientific articles written about it, perhaps because it is more expensive and less consumed.

Q: *I will be addressing white tea—a lot. What can you tell me that I may not know about it?*
A: Very little is known about the health effects of white tea. No human health studies have been published. However, I believe that studies with white tea would show similar health benefits to green tea.

Q: *Are there hundreds of antioxidant compounds in tea (black) and perhaps some we aren't even aware of? Please explain.*
A: Black tea has many unidentified compounds, not so for green and white tea. No human studies [conducted] with white tea.

Q: *Do you feel white tea will ever be more popular than green tea?*
A: No, because it is more expensive.

Q: *The major antioxidant in green tea is EGCG—what is it in white tea and black tea?*
A: ECGC is the major compound in white tea. I found an article that showed from the same cultivar that white tea had more of the individual polyphenols than green or black tea and that white tea polyphenols (flavonols) were more bioavailable (intestinal cells) than green or black tea.

So despite the different articles stating the amount of EGCG in white tea (it seems to depend on many factors), lack of groundbreaking, double-blind studies scrutinizing thousands of people—(currently, we only can see the results of lab rats and test tube studies)—we do know white tea does contain disease-fighting antioxidants like black and green tea. But the question is, exactly how healthy is white tea and just how good is it for you?

In the next chapter, I delve into the answers to the question: Is white tea the new green tea—or is it hopeful hype? But first, take a quick glance at the nutritional benefits that may help stave off health ailments and diseases—and in the next chapter I'll show you exactly how these nutrients of the rare tea give some credibility to its health benefits.

HEALING NUTRIENTS OF WHITE TEA

Drinking white tea brewed from loose leaves provides the most anti-oxidants because it has less processing than tea bags. Also, flavored white teas infused with spices, herbs, and fruits will provide extra nutrients and antioxidants, which give you more healing powers from head to toe.

The nutrients of white tea are plentiful but some of the main ones you should know about include: caffeine, catechins, epigallocatechin-3-gallate, flavonoids, fluoride, polyphenols, tannins, and theobromine. As noted in the first chapter on tea, these compounds are disease fighters.

That means white tea may help lower the risk of developing cancer, type 2 diabetes, heart disease, obesity, and dental caries. Also, as you'll discover in following chapters, while the fluoride is good for your teeth, white tea is often preferred over darker teas for a reason you may like. (Refer to chapter 18 to discover more about white tea and its benefits.)

One-Bowl Tea-Infused Rice with Vegetables

During lean times (and there were plenty of hard times throughout my twenties and thirties), I dined on a lot of rice and vegetables because it was fail-safe to make, cheap, and healthy. One night after classes and scrubbing floors and obliterating cobwebs, I was tired but hungry. My college roomie created a run-of-the-mill rice meal. He sautéed a variety of cruciferous vegetables and cooked a big pot of white rice. It fed more than eight of us. But now-adays, I know by adding tea, herbs, and spices, this dish can be even more tea-licious—rich or poor. Tea-infused rice and veggies can also enhance your health and well-being. This is my recipe inspired by college days gone better. A savory dish, like this one, is an introduction to the joy of tea cuisine. It's healthier than ordering Chinese takeout, and you're in charge of the ingredients, flavor, and presentation.

4 cups water
2 cups white rice, cooked
2 teaspoons Silver Needles white tea leaves (The Cozy
   Cart Tea)
2 cups fresh vegetable mix, washed (broccoli, carrots,
   snow peas, mushrooms, water chestnuts) chopped,
   or precut and packaged
2 tablespoons lemon extra virgin olive oil
1 teaspoon European-style butter
1 clove fresh garlic, minced
Ground pepper as desired
Sea salt to taste

Follow cooking rice instructions on the package using water and rice, but add tea to the mixture. While simmering, stir-fry vegetable mix in ingredients list in oil, butter, and garlic. Add pepper and salt. Top cooked rice with vegetables. Lightly toss. Serves 3–4. Brew a pot of white tea, such as White Peony or Silver Needle. (Refer to the next chapter. This type of tea is often served in Chinese restaurants.)

Almond Tea Cookies

Almond Tea Cookies (a light and favorite exotic treat to serve with a fresh pot of tea) seem to taste better homemade instead of store-bought. In fact, when I shared these with readers in a food column I wrote, I knew it worked because I was receiving orders for my Asian entrée and tea cookies! While that wasn't my plan, I can understand how nice it would be to receive a dinner-in-a-box with elegant cookies to pair with a pot of white tea for dinner guests or afternoon tea.

1½ cups 100 percent all-purpose flour
½ cup granulated sugar

½ teaspoon baking soda
Sea salt, a dash
½ cup Mediterranean-style butter
2 tablespoons organic half-and-half
1 brown egg
1½ teaspoons almond extract
½ cup ground almonds (chop in blender)

In a bowl, mix flour, sugar, baking soda, and salt. Cut in butter. Add half-and-half, beaten egg, extract, and almonds. Roll cookie dough mixture into ball. Chill for 30 minutes in the refrigerator. Roll into petite, 1-inch balls and place each one on parchment-lined cookie sheet. Press a sliced almond on top. Bake at 375 degrees for about 10 minutes or until light golden brown. Cool. Optional: Glaze with powdered sugar and milk (about ¼ cup each) and ¼ teaspoon pure vanilla extract. Makes approximately 16.

TEA-CENTRIC HEALING HINTS TO STEEP

✓ The ingredients most healing in white tea are the antioxidants.
✓ It's the antioxidant epigallocatechin-3-gallate (EGCG) that has been pinpointed as the major polyphenol player in *both* white and green teas.
✓ Do not ignore its antibacterial powers, which are in the brew as well as soaps and beauty products.
✓ White tea may never be as popular as black tea but serious tea drinkers who adore specialty teas will continue to drink this healing tea, increasing its demand.
✓ And millennials may gravitate toward the healing tea in tea blends and solo as a special tea to savor for its taste and healing powers.

Is White Tea Good for You?

*Thank God for tea! What would the world do
   without tea!
How did we exist! I am glad I was not born before
   tea!*
—Sydney Smith, *A Memoir of the Rev. Sydney Smith*

During my time spent on the coast of Southern California, my gran in the Southwestern desert was on my mind. Tea time—sharing the white-green tea paired with her homemade cookies during monsoon season—was the next destination. My mode of transportation was the typical seventies style—hitching and hiking to get through the 500-mile trek. Once I was out of Los Angeles, headed east on Highway 10, the congested city morphed into a wasteland. My clothes were glued to my body with sweat, and the ponytail that lay on the back of my neck was rapidly wilting. There was no sound in the desert except for the subtle buildup of a feverish breeze that whistled through the dry air.

As a car approached the on-ramp where I waited, I stuck out my thumb and watched the vehicle pass me. Instead of dwelling on the memory of the NO GAS-FOOD-LODGING 120 MILES sign, I attempted to sing a familiar tune.

An hour later a dilapidated pickup with two kids in the back stopped.

"I'm headed to Tucson," I said.

"We go, too," said the driver, a migrant worker. He flicked his head to tell me to get in the back of the vehicle. I threw my backpack into the truck and climbed in after it. The children made me smile and I sang for them. "Over the river and through the woods, to grand-mother's house we go . . ." from "The New-England Boy's Song about Thanksgiving Day." The children laughed at the funny lady who sang about Christmas and snow in the summer heat in the desert. But it made me feel cooler and I sang it all the way through twice. Then, the kids handed me a plastic pitcher from the ice chest. "Drink." It was cold sweet tea. I wasn't in California and I was far from the Southeast where this black tea and white sugar drink is popular, yet the swig I took made me feel at home in the middle of nowhere.

When I wrote *The Healing Powers of Vinegar*, I ran into a snag when discovering there were no human studies to prove red wine vinegar contained as much resveratrol as red wine—but one scientist did do research tests for me and discovered it indeed contained resveratrol. Similarly, not only are white tea's high amount of antioxidants good for preventing health ailments but it may just help lower the risk of developing specific diseases.

On the upside, white tea does have more research (even though we have to credit lab rats and petri dishes) than red wine vinegar, and def-initely more studies than balsamic vinegar, pointing to the promise of healing powers. Here are some words of wisdom from researchers to show you why white tea is often called the new green tea.

WHITE TEA AND MORE HEALTH VIRTUES

Take a closer look at the powers of white tea and perhaps if you in-clude it on your tea menu you may bypass these diseases through your lifetime. The good news is, we are learning that heart disease can be prevented, especially with a healthful diet and lifestyle. Cancer, how-ever, may end up being the number one killer in the future. Personally, I believe good genes and luck play a role, too, and it's important to begin with diet—and that includes tea—white tea.

Immune System: Since white tea, not unlike its counterpart black tea, boasts antibacterial properties, it can bolster the immune system. In other words, white tea can help to lower the risk of getting viruses like the flu, cold, and even cancer.

The key antioxidant in white tea is EGCG (discussed in previous chapters), which may help neutralize bad free radicals in your body's cells so it can keep cancer away. Researchers at Kingston University in London discovered the high polyphenols may even help keep your skin younger looking and healthier as well as reduce aging wrinkles. The positive results may be due to the enzymes in white tea that break down elastin and collagen which can trigger wrinkles.[1]

Heart Disease: The Ultimate Tea Diet authors Mark Ukra and Sharon Kolberg explain, "White teas and green teas have slightly higher levels of polyphenols (antioxidants found in plants); oolong and black tea have recently been shown to be more effective in preventing certain diseases, such as heart disease and high blood pressure." But the general consensus is that the kind of tea you drink is not as important as the fact that you drink it.[2]

White tea is an excellent heart-healthy tea because of its catechins (the good guys that can help lower cholesterol levels—the stuff that can clog your arteries). And it does contain less caffeine than black tea so some people are more prone to brew a cup of white tea in the afternoon for a pick-me-up energy boost rather than pass like they do on black tea.

Inflammation and Joints: Furthermore, white tea's higher level of antioxidants may help explain why it has been reported to help lessen inflammation and joint pain from rheumatoid arthritis (RA), a chronic inflammatory disorder that can affect your joints and other body systems. It is believed to be better than some green teas and may also have a positive effect on cholesterol levels linked to heart disease. While more research is needed, the study shows promise for white tea and its potential healing powers to enhance good health and longevity. And some medical researchers agree and tout both black and the rare white tea.[3]

As an ethical health journalist who will not sugarcoat or sensationalize the outcome of superfoods, I cannot promise you that drinking white tea is a magic bullet cure for cancer or will keep your ticker ticking until you're 120. But incorporating white tea—and other teas—

into a healthful diet and lifestyle may indeed help you live a healthier life.

When I interviewed tea expert Jeffrey Blumberg, Ph.D., I was anticipating some super words on the superfood white tea. Well, I did get the thumbs-up on tea—but not one type. Keep in mind, drinking the main tea types—black, white, green, and oolong—and herbal teas can help you stay healthier. And white tea blends are definitely something to consider adding to your tea menu—including foods like a healthful smoothie.

White Tea and Strawberry Smoothie

½ cup organic 2% low-fat milk
½ cup white tea, brewed, cooled
1 cup vanilla honey Greek yogurt
1 cup fresh strawberries, sliced, frozen
4 ice cubes
2 teaspoons pure vanilla extract
2 tablespoons wheat germ
Whipped cream (optional) for garnish

In blender, mix milk, tea, yogurt, and berries. Add ice cubes and vanilla. Blend. Sprinkle wheat germ on top and blend a few seconds. Top with whipped cream. Serves 2.

In the next chapter, you'll be departing the visit to the world of white tea as I take you to a more familiar place—green tea. Years ago, I was hired by a medical doctor to edit a book on green tea. I found that studies abounded (including ones on green tea extract) and were fascinating, despite my fondness for black tea, which I sipped while nurturing his green tea book. While you find out how green tea varieties can help you healthy up, take a look at both chapter 14 and chapter 15 on anti-aging and skinny teas (green tea is included) for information that'll wow you about how an assortment of teas—not just green—can help you stay younger longer and keep unwanted pounds and body fat at bay.

TEA-CENTRIC HEALING HINTS TO STEEP

✓ Aging   Polyphenols and antibacterial compounds help to slow down the effects of aging inside and outside the body, face, skin.

✓ Cancer   Antioxidants in white tea help lower the risk of of developing lung and skin cancer.

✓ Diabetes   Compounds in white tea help manage unsteady sugar levels.

✓ High blood pressure Potassium in white tea helps lessen heart problems.

✓ Overweight   Caffeine in white tea aids in weight loss.

PART 4

OTHER TEA TYPES

Healthy Green Tea

*All true tea lovers not only like their tea strong,
but like it a little stronger with each year that
passes.*
—"A Nice Cup of Tea," by George Orwell,
in the *Evening Standard*, January 12, 1946

After my journey to the Southwest, I hitched and hiked back to the West Coast, where tea played a role again in providing vim and vigor. En route to the Golden State, at truck stops and roadside cafés, small metal tea kettles and black tea kept me alert at night; a reminder of my roots in San Jose—a place where iced tea with lemon slices were "the" beverage in the hot summer. After a short visit I was on the road with my dog, Stone Fox. Northbound, I ended up in Eugene, Oregon, a place where young people flocked and lived a natural lifestyle. One night in the company of a young couple with an upscale hippie vibe living in an inviting house (it seemed like a mansion out of the *Howards End* film) I was introduced to a different tea—green tea. I felt awkward like the film's character Leonard Bast when sitting down to a perfect display of tea and scones.

The woman was an inspiration to me: Her indoor garden with a plant light, two kittens, stereo, and vast tea collection (loose leaves labeled in individual packets like a science) opened up a new world to me. In the nighttime she offered me a cup of tea (which was straight out of the dark setting in the food and tea scene in *The Hobbit: An Unexpected Journey*). She served a cup of strong green tea. I tasted a sweet flowerlike beverage paired with clover honey and a bowl of fresh blackberries. Like Goldilocks, seeking the perfect bed, I had found the perfect cup of tea. I experienced an epiphany that night: For some inexplicable reason I wanted to learn more about tea—all tea types—not just black, white, and green. There had to be more. And decades later, here I am in the land of teas including green tea.

I was not alone in my interest in the brew. Medical studies (especially with green tea extract) became popular in the late 20th century and into the early 21st century. It is not my favorite tea, though, despite my past in Oregon, I confess I sipped black tea and herbal teas more in my past and present-day. Green tea has made its way into my tea cupboard but in blends like a green and white tea specialty cup I ordered in Vancouver, British Columbia's former hot spot The Urban Tea Merchant.

THE GREEN HISTORY OF GREEN TEA

While green tea may have been introduced to me in the early 21st century, as legend tells it, it's been around for a long, long time. The *Tea Classic* book penned by Lu Yu during the Tang dynasty is a historical milestone and tribute to green tea. Later, the book *The Kissa Yojok Book of Tea*, created by Zen priest Eisai in the late 12th century, notes the healing powers of green tea and how it influences the human body. But green tea doesn't end there . . .

Fast-forward to America in the 20th century and history shows that before World War II (before the conflict between Japan and China), green tea was the most popular variety in the United States. Of course, after the war, black tea moved in as the number one most consumed tea in America, and it still is in the 21st century.

GREEN TEA STAYS IN VOGUE

Since the late 20th century and into the 21st, green teas have been newly embraced for their variety of healing powers, despite the teas' roots going back to ancient history. "The health benefits and availability of green teas have kept it in vogue," points out Tea Master Daniel Johnson. "The informed contemporary tea drinker has learned to move beyond the mechanically processed green tea bag," he says. "They appreciate and love to drink loose tea selections of Sencha, pearl jasmine, and fine needle green tea."

However, green tea—and its varied types—wasn't always easily available. Twenty years ago, according to the Tea Association of the U.S.A., Inc., green tea was nearly impossible to find at your friendly supermarket. These days, green tea is a household name, especially on the West Coast, East Coast, in big U.S. cities, and in Asian countries. It can be found in grocery stores and stand-alone shops, online, in restaurants, and in luxury hotels.

Black tea—still the most popular tea in the United States—and white tea (rare but good and gaining in its good tea reputation) are two superstar teas in this book. Of course, I'm including healing green tea but it's not my focus as it has been for so many, from authors of tea books to scientists conducting tea and health studies.

While the nutrition facts for green tea are similar to analyzing vinegars (not a lot to see for a teaspoon of vinegar or one cup of brewed tea on a nutrition label), this tea type does contain trace amounts of vitamins and minerals. And note, with popular green tea, not unlike popular apple cider vinegar, the bigger the measurements, the more nutrients you'll find.

More Tea, Please

Tea (green), brewed, prepared with tap water; 3.5 ounces contains:

    0.96 calories
    0 g from total carbohydrate
    0 from fat
    0.2 from protein
    0.007 mg thiamine (B1)
    0.006 mg riboflavin
    0.03 mg niacin (B3)
    0.005 mg vitamin B6
    0.3 mg from vitamin C

0.02 mg iron
1 mg magnesium
0.18 manganese
8 mg potassium
1 mg sodium
Other constituents
99.9 water

Apparently, more tea equals more nutrients. One cup contains more good-for-you vitamins and minerals, water, and caffeine.

(*Source:* USDA SR-21 National Nutrient Database for Standard Reference)

So one cup of green tea—like one cup of black tea (as I've already noted, it's still the most favorite of all types of tea)—may look like it doesn't really have that much to offer when it comes to its ingredients list. But if you include its antioxidants then you've got something to hold on to for your health's sake and say regularly, "More, tea please" or "Yes, I'll have a second cup."

ANTIOXIDANTS: THE REAL HEALING POWER OF GREEN TEA

Green tea leads the pack in flavonoids between four tea varieties but white tea ranks second in EGCG, which is important in helping to lower risk of many diseases. Here, take a look:

FLAVONOIDS IN TEA TYPES

Tea Type	ECG	EGCG
Black Tea	5.9	9.4
White Tea	8.3	42.4
Oolong Tea	6.3	34.5
Green Tea	17.9	70.2

A typical cup of tea in Japan contains 3½ ounces. The total flavonoid content in green and black tea is about 138 mg and 118 mg per 3½ ounces. The catechins—a major subclass of flavonoids found in tea—include EGCG (epigallocatechin gallate).[1]

And it's time to take a close-up look at some popular green tea types and note the health benefits of each one.

GREEN TEA IS A DISEASE FIGHTER

In the 21st century, heart disease and cancer are the two culprits that affect our health, well-being, and lifespan. There is no cure for either but you can lower your risk of developing these diseases with diet and lifestyle—and that's where tea comes into play.

Heart Disease: Green tea's role in heart health is a big one. Past research in the noteworthy Ohsaki study published in the *Journal of the American Medical Association* (a peer-reviewed medical journal) discovered that 40,000 middle-aged men and women in Japan who drank about two cups of green tea each day reduced their risk of cardiovascular disease by a whopping 22 to 33 percent, compared to those who drank less than a half cup of green tea daily. The findings show without a shadow of doubt green tea plays a significant role in staying heart healthy.[2]

Cancer: Green tea, like white tea, contains EGCG (epigallocatechin gallate, a catechin, a class of polyphenols I mention time after time in this book and other books in the *Healing Powers* series). Researchers believe EGCG in green tea (and other superfoods) may inhibit the growth of cancers (and may help protect against heart disease) in different parts of the body and shows promise.

Instead of lists of lab studies that used green tea to study the EGCG, the key is that yes, tea's catechin in green tea does appear to put it in the cancer-fighting foods list. Still, more research is needed before the National Cancer Institute and American Cancer Society give green tea a stamp of approval for being a cancer fighter. So, until we have a definitive blessing from organizations like these, medical doctors, scientists, nutritionists, and tea companies, big and small, will not dish the statement "green tea *can* prevent cancer" because there still isn't enough cause and effect to prove that green tea is a cure-all.

A GARDEN VARIETY OF GREEN TEA TYPES

Green tea usually comes from Japan and China—two countries where this type of tea is popular and cancer incidence is lower than it is in the United States. Here are some of the most popular types to share with you and provide their healing benefits.

Dragon Well: Welcome to one of China's most popular green teas. Dragon Well is a mild yellow-colored tea with earthy sweetness. As a green tea, it is believed by medical researchers that it may help lower your risk of developing cancer, but as noted earlier, more research is needed.

Gunpowder: Grown in Zhanjang, this green tea is robust in flavor. It is popular, dark in color, and provides a distinct, smoky type of tea. Because of its extra caffeine content it's energizing for mind and body. No blessings needed here. All you have to do is drink a cup of gunpowder tea and you'll get the boost of motivation to enhance brainpower or exercise.

Jasmine: Not a green tea itself, it has a green tea base combined with white tea and black tea (as I explained in a past chapter when I tried my first cup of jasmine tea). It has a subtle, sweet fragrance. It is a popular tea in China and grows there as well as Vietnam and Japan.

Matcha: A powdered green tea from China and Japan, it has a strong and sweet distinct flavor that requires an acquired taste. Once you enjoy the taste you can enjoy its antioxidants, which are amazing according to both tea proponents and medical studies. Matcha contains L-theanine, a compound that is a feel-good de-stressor. (See chapter 18 to find out about why matcha and its reputation may have been affected after a Japanese natural disaster in 2011—and what you can do before ordering.)

Travels with a Tea Master: Great Vibrations

Daniel Johnson, not unlike other worldy tea masters, has toured faraway lands, including Asia, to experience the exotic side of tea and tea people. He shares in his own words a memorable event that occurred in China and paints a vivid picture of what may have been one of the best days of his life. . . .

Traveling from the city of Chengdu in Southern China, we drove hours passing valleys of terraced tea fields. Our destination was a temple at the top of Mount Emei. We spent three days hiking to the peak. Along our path we were able to rest and refresh our spirits at Taoist temples and kitchens along the mountains. Here we would drink fresh tea and eat dumplings while observing monkeys and the pristine beauty of the mountains.

On the second day, my two friends and I stopped for tea and dinner at a temple called the Elephants' Wading Pool. Despite not speaking Chinese we had gained success at ordering green tea and noodle soups. After we took off our backpacks and ordered our meal, I could not reduce my body temperature. I felt confined, hot, and claustrophobic sitting in the small earthen building. I walked over toward the wall and opened a window to invite a cool mountain breeze to refresh the air of the warm, stuffy room. Sitting down for a wonderful pot of green tea, I mistakenly invited more than a cool breeze into the small building.

Two monkeys climbed in through the window and began moving around the restaurant. Making a racket the intruding monkeys alerted one of the monks who was preparing our meal. The man, wrapped in a modest robe, grabbed a broom from the room corner and began to use his makeshift kung fu staff to clear the hungry monkeys from the room. After securing the open window, he glanced at me, and returned to the kitchen. The looks my companions and I shared over that pot of tea were priceless.

GRATEFUL TO THE GREEN TEA GARDENS

As a longtime San Francisco Bay Area resident and San Francisco State University alumna, it would be unforgivable for me not to have toured the tea gardens that go back in time to the 1800s. In my twenties, I was a graduate student, struggling to make ends meet. One day, in need of getting balanced, I went to Japanese Tea Garden, a popular attraction of Golden Gate Park and near the University of San Francisco's Student Union.

I was served a green tea (it was my second time after the Oregonian brew). During the tea ceremony I focused on the obstacles in my life. I rejoiced in a garden full of paths, ponds, plants, and trees. While sipping a calming cup of green tea (it was probably Sencha), I put the challenges into perspective while trying to savor the moment. In hindsight, I get it. Monks can stay relaxed and mindful when drinking tea and meditating. What's more, my mind was clear. I gained strength to move forward. I was grateful to the gardens and the tea ritual, which helped me to learn how to let go and go with the flow. It was tea and the ritual of regrouping that helped me find the answer.

It's no secret that green tea has been the "in" tea used in medical studies and tea books and for good reason. While basic green tea or exotic tea types can attract tea lovers, flavored green teas are definitely worth a mention. While green tea is not my number one favorite, I admit I was eager to try this tea—and yes, it is yummy, not to forget its health benefits. (I do not add milk or sugar to my tea for health's sake.) I tried Pomegranate Gem (from The Cozy Tea Cart)—with Sencha from China as the green tea base with rose petals. I whipped up a Green Tea Pomegranate Lemonade for one: 1 teaspoon tea leaves, 1 cup hot water, ¼ cup all-natural lemonade, ice cubes, lemon slices for garnish. Not only did I get my dose of antioxidants—the iced tea was an enjoyable green tea creation. Another surprise: Another type of green tea is available that you may not be aware of, nor was I. . . .

INTRODUCING RARE YELLOW TEA

Yellow tea is considered a rare tea by tea masters and for good reason. Like white tea, yellow tea is not that plentiful and only found in China. Actually, it's lesser known than white tea but it may have the same healing powers as both green and white teas. It's not surprising that because of its low profile medical studies are not abundant but that doesn't mean it's not worth your while to become familiar with this specialty tea. Yellow tea, like other teas, contains antioxidants that can stave off inflammation, which scientists believe may be the culprit behind many life-threatening diseases.

Matcha Tea Ice Cream

Rather than make your own ice cream from scratch or turn to a store-bought brand of quality tea-infused matcha ice cream like Häagen-Dazs (it is good), why not try a semi-homemade recipe? This way, matcha powder is from a source of your choice as is quality ice cream—your favorite brand. And by mixing the green powder into the fresh ice cream (you can use Greek yogurt, too) it feels like you're putting more tender loving care into it than buying it pre-made. Plus, you can pair the matcha ice cream with one of the tea cookies you do make from scratch. (Find recipes in chapter 20, "Tea Menu".) Also, by making a semi-homemade ice cream (if you have the time and knack bring out the ice cream maker like the chefs do on the Food Network) you'll have more time to make tea cookies (the aroma will linger in the kitchen), add fresh fruit, nuts, and brew a good pot of tea (I recommend black or white).

1 pint premium vanilla ice cream
*½–1 teaspoon matcha powder (I prefer a lighter green
    color, which looks more appetizing)*
½ cup almonds, chopped
2 cups fresh fruit, chopped
Whipped cream, real (optional)

Let ice cream soften in carton at room temperature. In a bowl, mix in matcha powder. Fold in nuts. Freeze until firm. Top with fresh fruit. Add a dollop of whipped cream. Serves 4.

Now that I've put green tea on the table, I feel I can move forward and introduce you to red tea—it is my goal to decode this tea for me, you, and your health's sake. Red tea is getting a lot of head turns in the 21st century, and in the next chapter you'll find out why.

TEA-CENTRIC HEALING HINTS TO STEEP

✓ Like its cousins black tea and white tea, green tea comes from the *Camellia sinensis* plant. Medical doctors and researchers will tell you these teas have similar healing powers, but they also seem to have different attributes, especially if you are looking for differences.

✓ Using green tea by drinking it or applying it topically has many health benefits noted in medical research *and* anecdotal evidence; the biggest health benefit buzz is that it may help lower the risk of developing cancers—but since the jury is still out it's up to you to make it your cup of tea . . .

✓ And like black tea, green tea (leaves, bags, and matcha) may help guard against heart disease due to its plentiful antioxidants.

✓ Green tea may be a dieter's aid by burning stored fat and boosting calorie-burning power.

The Red Tea Boom

The scattered tea goes with the leaves and every day a sunset dies.
  —William Faulkner, *As I Lay Dying*

As serendipity would have it, the Oregonian couple needed a house sitter for one week; I desired a place to stay and regroup. I was spooked by the back-to-nature lifestyle, but indulged. Not accustomed to the cold climate, I thought: "Tea will warm me up." But I had to chop firewood for the only source of heat: a wood-burning stove. Not only did cutting my finger with an ax put me in alarm mode, but I was also catching a cold while acknowledging I wasn't a hardy mountain woman; I'd rather be sitting in a Victorian tearoom drinking red tea and enjoying crumpets. I viewed the canned soup collection; but I needed more of a rescue effort than tomato soup.

Looking at the inventory of her tea cupboard, I read the white stick-on DIY labels with her printed words. I picked up one and read: "Hibiscus: Vitamin C." That was the herbal tea I chose. The loose leaves turned an orange-red when I poured it into a glass tea mug; I took my tea to the loft and climbed into bed with my canine companion, Stone Fox, as we broke the "no dog in bed" house rules. My black Lab kept me cozy all night long, not unlike the tea I sipped and savored.

In the morning when I awoke, my index finger throbbed, thanks to my poor wood-chopping skills. I didn't know how to work the plant light, and the house was cold again. I stoked a new fire, and brewed another cup of the red drink. I wanted to learn more about the land of tea. I'll now share with you more information about red tea—real red tea.

DECODING RED TEA

The phenomenon of red tea can be a tea ball strainer of confusion. Blame the different types of tea and tisanes with a mix of red-orange hues on the mix-up, as well as the differences between Eastern and Western cultures. So, it's time to provide clarity on the red tea boom— from herbal rooibos to red tea—once and for all.

Red tea, tea proponents will tell you, is a term for a reddish-colored tea—with roots that lead back to black tea in China centuries ago. It is linked to what we in the West call "black tea." Hong cha, or "red tea," is the authentic name for black tea and it is called this in the East because in Asia, teas are often named simply for the color of the liquid. The confusion about the red tea phenomenon doesn't stop there. . . .

OOLONG TEA, THE ORANGE-REDDISH BREW

Now we have black tea *and* oolong tea that once brewed can be red in color. And so, let me get you settled in with oolong tea. Unlike red tisanes (hibiscus, red clover, and rooibos), oolong tea is a real tea with Asian roots. Oolong (called Black Dragon because when in a teapot it resembles the shape of a dragon) is a Chinese and Taiwanese tea with a fruity scent. The first time I was introduced to this red tea was when I called a Chinese restaurant in San Carlos, California—it had been my favorite go-to for a sit-down dinner or takeout. Since the town I'd lived in for 15 years morphed due to gentrification, it was no surprise the eatery had changed its owners—and choice of tea. No longer was jasmine or green tea served—it was oolong, the server on the phone told me. She said: "It's reddish-orange tea color." And that was my first taste of one of the main varieties of tea.

The second event of oolong tea entering my life was when reading health guru Jonny Bowden's words that all four kinds of non-herbal tea including oolong (red)—come from the same plant, *Camellia sinen-*

sis. He doesn't expound on the red tea, most likely because it's not as popular as black tea and green tea.[1]

In my tea pantry I found an assortment of the red tea behind the black, white, and herbal teas. These included Oolong Tea White Peach Stash Tea, Bigelow Oolong Tea, and Choice Oolong. To me these teas called out for iced tea infused with fresh summer fruit, like lemons and oranges, in the clear pitcher that sits on a kitchen shelf. If you do research on this Chinese tea, you'll discover as I did that it is a semi-oxidized tea and comes from the Fujian province. Like black, white, and green teas, it does contain disease-fighting antioxidants. That means it's the polyphenols (good-for-you antioxidants found in superfoods discussed in previous chapters) in this red tea that may help guard against cancer and heart diseases.

ROOIBOS, THE NON-TEA RISING

Hello again, rooibos (*Aspalathus linearis*), pronounced (roy-boss), a red tea grown only in South Africa. In the West, the common definition for red tea is rooibos, which is an herbal tea. Its roots go way back to the early 1700s, thanks to a Swede named Carl Thumberg, who observed that the tea came from a red bush. He noted the mountain people would cut the leaves from rooibos plants, dried in the sun, and concoct red tea as a beverage.

In my tea cupboard in the dining-kitchen area, I know there are tea blends with rooibos but while this tea does contain many healing properties, it is not my first choice. Yet the more I discover data about rooibos, it makes me wonder why I don't give it more attention, as other tea researchers do.

Peter Goggi of the Tea Association of the U.S.A. tells me, "When brewed, its appearance mimics that of black tea in color, but bears no relation to black tea in the areas of taste, aroma, and antioxidant properties. In comparison to black tea (or green, white, oolong, and dark teas)," he adds, "there are far fewer peer-reviewed studies regarding any health benefits." We both agree it appears sellers of rooibos tout its healing powers, "but most of the claims are anecdotal in nature, and very few clinical studies have been published, as compared to *Camellia sinesis*," points out Goggi.

Some tea authorities, like sellers, claim it is the "new" herbal tea on the block—in America, that is. It's been used around the world for over 200 years. In the nineties, I recall one tea authority praising rooibos as the new healing wonder. Since it wasn't familiar to me, I ignored the words and focused on other herbal teas.

But then, later on in the 21st century—it's déjà vu as I face the red tea boom. Tea people tell me that like green tea and black tea, rooibos contains "powerful antioxidants" that make this "non-tea" good for heart health and the immune system just like real teas. So, can this herbal red tea enhance your health and turn back the clock and boost your longevity?

Not unlike black, white, and green teas, if you look at a nutritional label on a basic box of tea bags you'll find something similar to this nutritional information:

NUTRITIONAL INFORMATION OF ROOIBOS TEA

This chart dishes basic nutrients for rooibos tea (traditional and green rooibos). Rooibos does not contain fat and is very low in sodium, caffeine-free, and a source of antioxidants. [SARC website, 2016: B]

	Per 100 ml tea
Energy (kJ)	0
Protein	0
Glycaemic carbohydrate (g) of which total	0
Sugar (g)	0
Total fat (g) of which saturated fat (g)	0
Dietary fiber (g)	0
Total sodium (mg)	3.8

(*Source:* Provided by the South African Rooibos Council based on analysis at SANAS-accredited laboratories)

But that's not all. . . .

MORE PROOF OF LIFE IN ROOIBOS TEA

Like the basic antioxidant-rich teas, rooibos, another healthy brew, contains a plentiful blend of antioxidants. Take a look at its round-up of antioxidants, shared by the South African Rooibos Council.

- Rooibos is the only known source of a specifically beneficial and rare antioxidant called aspalathin.
- Unfermented (green) rooibos has higher levels of antioxidants than traditional, fermented rooibos.
- The antioxidants in rooibos are potent enough to measurably elevate the antioxidant levels in blood, thereby boosting the body's internal defense systems against disease. The effect peaks about one hour after drinking 500 ml rooibos tea.
- The antioxidant content of rooibos also depends on the soil conditions of the region where the plant was grown, and how the infusion was prepared.

Past research has pinpointed more than dozens of polyphenols in red tea. These compounds act as disease fighters that are capable of destroying free radicals in the body. This depletes the immune system and makes it more prone to diseases, including inflammatory conditions such as arthritis, heart disease, and cancer. And red tea like rooibos may help your body to fight back.

Other researchers have discovered rooibos not only contains polyphenols, including flavanols and flavanones—but also quercetin, a "super antioxidant" that is excellent for the immune system. Quercetin can act as a natural antihistamine and inhibit histamine release from mast cells (cells that produce histamine). It is also touted as an anti-cancer antioxidant and is found in onion as well as rooibos.[2]

What's more, unlike caffeinated teas, herbal tea rooibos does not contain caffeine and has fewer tannins than black tea or green tea. Plus, the immunity aid of the vitamin C content in this herbal tea is something to write home about, especially since it can be good for you during stressful times when antioxidants can keep you healthy, and during cold and flu season. Because of its multiple healing components, it's used in many herbal blends as well as white tea.

To enjoy a cup of rooibos (it can be served both hot or iced as is or in a blend)—place 1 tea bag or 1 rounded teaspoon of loose tea leaves in an 8-ounce cup. Add boiling water. Steep at least 3 minutes. This quick DIY recipe will get you started and eager to go to tea companies offering rooibos and rooibos tea blends, including Harney & Sons and The Cozy Tea Cart, Numi, and Bigelow. It is a reddish color and has a sweet, woodsy, earthy flavor that is similar to some black teas I've sipped. Also, rooibos is used in fruity dessert teas and masala chai blends. But wait, there are more red teas to share.

ENTER MORE RED TEAS

Meet hibiscus (*Hibiscus rosa-sinensis*), an herbal tea that is rich in vitamin C—a vitamin used to boost the immune system and help stave off colds, flus, and cancers. This vitamin is also known to be the anti-stress vitamin of choice. Hibiscus is used in a variety of herbal tea and flavored tea blends because of its sweet flavor, as well as its wellness potential.

WILD FLOWER HIBISCUS EXTRAORDINAIRE

As one who is an herbal tea fan, I'm surprised that I didn't know a lot about hibiscus until I had a chance to grill the man behind the flower that is blossoming in the land of tisanes. As the story goes, Wild Hibiscus Flower Company director Chris Muir began making native Australian jams with quandong, Riberry, and other indigenous products from the Australian outback. Rosella, which is what Australians call hibiscus, was one of the jams. And the rest is history. Let me share some of the gems straight from the man himself. . . .

Q: *Tell me more about rosella.*
A: Tart like a cranberry, it is a fairly common jam for mothers and grandmothers to make for their families. In the outback on farms, it is common to be part of the produce grown; the tough little rosella bushes will survive strong heat as long as they have a little water each day. My mother would make her rosella jam each year and my father would add a spoonful or two to his vanilla ice cream that very night, one of his favorite things to do and he still does it. From making jams, our company founder, Lee Etherington, figured out a natural way to

preserve our flowers whole, which led to the flagship Wild Hibiscus product sold around the world, Wild Hibiscus Flowers in Syrup. As a way to keep all areas of our company running in a sustainable fashion it was then a natural extension to create a hibiscus tea to use any flowers that were too big or small for our flagship product.

Q: *The popularity of red teas confuses people like me! Clarify the confusion of the varieties of red tea—and why do you sell hibiscus instead of rooibos?*

A: Teas are relative to the region in the world they are from, just like the culture they are part of. Popular enough or discovered by other regions around the world or if there are trade issues for another tea product, the new alternative is then exported or imported around the world, and so begins the education process and the new tea is added to the bountiful basket of options. When you account for all of this discovery and trade around the world, an enthusiast, just like a wine connoisseur, has so much to learn and experience about the many varieties, blends, and styles that are available.

Hibiscus is common in many parts of the world, from Africa to the Middle East, Asia, and the Americas. In each part of the world it is used in different ways culturally: in Egypt as the wedding toast, in Mexico a deliciously well-balanced cold beverage consumed by all ages, in Australia in jam or as a tea or as a garnish.

The hibiscus we know was most likely brought down from tribes or seafarers millennia ago to Australia, but we consider it part of our traditions, so this is why we use hibiscus. Rooibos is from South Africa and its usage dates back to the tribes of the Cederberg region using it. A little study on the history of it, a little tasting of the many varieties available . . . a rooibos compared to a hibiscus tea is very different so there is little confusion.

Q: *Do you personally drink this tea and for what healing reason has it helped you?*

A: Yes, usually a cup every night. I find that with my busy lifestyle one can get a little run-down. If I do not consume a cup of hibiscus every night or second night, in the past I have noticed I am more likely to pick up a cold or bug, or feel a little more run-down. For an added boost I like to combine a sachet of our butterfly pea flower tea with hibiscus; the pH of the hibiscus changes the blue tea to a very pretty purple. In addition, butterfly pea has an ORAC rating of 7022 per cup of tea. As an alternative to a hot beverage, for my three children, we will make healthy red Popsicles during the summer from our hibiscus tea (add a natural sweetener before freezing). Very easy and they love it!

Chocolate Chip Pancakes with a Pot of Oolong Tea

Chocolate, pancakes, and tea all have something in common: They are comfort foods—and they can be served and savored year-round. This recipe is mine and inspired by the charming film *Something's Gotta Give* (2003), when two seniors played by actors Diane Keaton and Jack Nicholson (dealing with health issues/aging and romance) want to enjoy pancakes for a late-night snack. Flapjacks can be made from scratch and served for breakfast, brunch, or any time—like superfoods dark chocolate and tea. Also, pairing red tea with chocolate works well and you'll get a double punch of disease-fighting antioxidants.

1 cup all-purpose flour
1 teaspoon baking powder
¾ cup organic 2% reduced fat milk (or buttermilk)
1½ tablespoons European-style butter
1 organic brown egg
1 capful pure vanilla extract
2 teaspoons rooibos tea (dried leaves, lightly or finely ground)
½ cup chocolate chips (dark or milk)
Butter to taste
Pure organic maple syrup (or honey)
Confectioners' sugar (optional)
1 cup fresh berries

In a bowl, mix flour, baking powder, milk, butter, and egg. Add vanilla and tea. Fold in chocolate chips. On medium heat, pour batter (⅓–½ cup ice cream scoop size) into frying pan. When the pancakes bubble, flip. Serve with a small pat of butter, syrup or honey, a sprinkle of confectioners' sugar, and seasonal berries. Serves approximately 5–6 small pancakes.

So, as you can see, red tea is a complicated tea ball of tea and tisanes when you include the concepts of East and West for black tea; oolong tea with its reddish-orange color; rooibos, the tisane that continues to get credit for its medicinal properties; and not to forget other "red" berry non-teas, which I've included in the next chapter on healing herbal teas. These will be found in the fruit tea section because they seemed to fit nicely all together in any season—winter, spring, fall, or summer.

TEA-CENTRIC HEALING HINTS TO STEEP

✓ Red tea is a term used for many teas and tisanes—East black tea and West rooibos—which may be the root of its confusion.
✓ Red tea includes rooibos, and to many tea proponents is more powerful than real teas because of the immune-enhancing perks of its vitamin C, as well as its disease-fighting antioxidants.
✓ Specialty teas include unique and single origin rooibos teas with different flavors, and medicinal benefits come with the package. Not to forget rooibos tea blends, which are plentiful and popular.
✓ Rooibos gained its popularity back in the late 20th century and it's still paving the way in the herbal tea parade.

1 1

Healing Herbal Teas

Tea is a divine herb.
—Xu Guangqi

I left bittersweet memories in Oregon to enroll in college at San Francisco, a city where I found a sense of belonging—and my cup of tea on and off campus. It was at the student union and nearby café that took me to the place where I fell in love with the world of non-teas or so-called herbal teas and tisanes. One memorable afternoon, at the student union, I ordered ginseng tea—it gave me a boost of mental energy to get me through the next class—Creative Writing in the afternoons to the D-day of my oral exams.

I was edgy after studying for months. The challenging task was to be tested on three authors of my choice (George Eliot, Edward Albee, and John Steinbeck); and to be grilled about their works and lives by a panel—a trio of no-nonsense English professors. It was chamomile tea (and imagining the professors were toy poodles I was training) that calmed me through this three-hour session that would determine if I'd attain a master's degree. The tea-related words of Eleanor Roosevelt are fitting: "A woman is like a tea bag—you can't tell how strong she is until you put her in hot water." Thanks to herbal tea I survived the challenge and passed my oral exams.

HERBAL TEA HAVEN

Here, take a look at popular herbal tea varietals that I've tasted and enjoyed throughout the years from the West Coast to the East Coast and Canada (a place where Red Rose tea—orange pekoe—is popular). Keep in mind, herbal teas are not considered "teas" because they do not come from the same plant as real teas, such as black tea and white tea do. Tisanes or "non-teas" come from different parts of a plant, including bark, flowers, leaves, roots, seeds, and stems.

There are hundreds of unique types of herbal teas available around the world. While herbal teas do not contain caffeine, they do contain other health-boosting ingredients that can do your body and mind a world of good. Herbal tea vendors, tea lovers, and health-conscious people of all ages are quick to tell you the healing powers of tisanes are infinite as well as the aromas and flavors. Enjoying both teas and tisanes is like having the best of both worlds. The more you widen your love for variety, the more healing rewards you may reap.

Herbal teas go way back in time. For centuries, people have been reaping the rewards of the vast variety of herbal teas. One of the benefits I like is that the color and flavor of herbal teas, often but not always, is more delicate than those of black or dark teas. Their heavenly scents and flavors offer you another way to enjoy the healing powers of non-teas.

In the Mediterranean diet and lifestyle, herbs and spices are part of the food pyramid, which makes sense. In fact, in European countries, single herbal teas are enjoyed: think lavender and chamomile. In the United States, however, in the 21st century tea companies offer us a great variety of special blends of herbs mixed with spices and fruits. There are so many types it's like being a child in an ice cream store trying to choose which one to try. Also, during each season you'll notice the different blends continue to grow and lure you to befriend the new herbal tea for the thrill and healing powers of it all. And herbal teas are "generally" safe for children, says Dr. Fred Pescatore, M.D., a well-known New York–based doctor and author who specializes in natural medicine, including children's disorders. "However," he points out, "there are certain herbal teas that aren't herbal at all but more medicinal." So, tisanes like chamomile and lemon balm are safe for kids, adds the good doctor, but wellness teas like valerian root aren't good or meant for kids. "If it is fruit tea or ginger tea those are good and far better than any energy drinks or soda."

Take a look at the wide variety of herbal historical highlights, health benefits, different ways to brew a perfect cuppa, and the Health Check pointers. (These are safety precautions and notes for *possible* side effects.) Follow up and go to chapter 18—discover alternative options for tisanes, so you can have your tea, so to speak, and drink it, too. Also, some of these herbal teas can be paired with teas in healing blends for better results.

CALENDULA (*Calendula officinalis*): A yellow flower used in an herbal tea brew is not unlike chamomile and is an herbal delight that I experienced by surprise. When I was introduced to an herbal blend, calendula was in it. Calendula is used as a digestive aid as well as topically for skin inflammation—not unlike chamomile. *Tisane Time:* Use in a blend with chamomile for best results.

CATNIP (*Nepeta cataria*): This herb (not your cat's plaything) is one like calendula that I discovered in tea blends, but goes back thousands of years and was praised for its multiple powers. Enjoyed by Europeans before it arrived in Asian countries, it boasts wide-ranging healing powers. Because of its properties, catnip can help in calming anxiety by relaxing the nervous system. The first time I was introduced to this herb was in a blend of catnip, calendula, linden flowers, and chamomile. *Tisane Time:* Put 1 tea bag of this blend or 1 teaspoon of the herb in one cup of hot water. Let it steep for 5 minutes. *Health Check:* If pregnant or trying to conceive, this may not be the right herbal tea for you.

Chamomile Secrets That'll Surprise You

CHAMOMILE (*Matricaria chamomilla*): Sweet Chamomile is my number-one favorite brew year-round and has been for years—despite the wide array of non-teas sitting in my tea cupboard. I love chamomile tea for its effects on my mind, body, and spirit, and the memories I have of drinking it while reading Emily Dickinson's love poems in the springtime amid the blossoming trees in the Santa Cruz Mountains.

Chamomile tea (a mainstay in my diet regime, both bags and loose leaf) goes back more than 2,000 years. A daisy-like plant found in both the United States and Europe, it has been considered a medicinal miracle, known as "ground apple" by the Greeks because of its fragrant scent. The Egyptians believed it to be sacred to the sun god Ra. In ancient Europe, chamomile petals were crushed to make soothing teas.

It is the herbal tea of choice to relax and sleep like a baby—or bunny. Remember *The Tale of Peter Rabbit* by Beatrix Potter? After Peter's big adventure, his mother put him to bed with a cup of chamomile for sweet dreams.

Researchers also believe that drinking chamomile tea can boost urine levels of glycine, a compound that relaxes muscle spasms or even menstrual cramps. Chamomile contains anti-inflammatory ingredients, so it's no wonder it can shrink hemorrhoids—and putting a wet chamomile tea bag on each eye can reduce puffiness, too. Not only does calming chamomile contain glycine, it also has other vitamins and minerals that provide the wow factor.

And it's no surprise that drinking several cups of chamomile tea weekly may add years to your lifespan, according to researchers from the University of Texas Medical Branch at Galveston. Findings show chamomile tea may lower the risk of death from all causes in older women by about 30 percent. The scientists of the published study in the *Gerontologist* point to the anti-immunity boosting effects, which may be one reason why it may stall Father Time. But more research is needed. Meanwhile, I will still continue to relish my chamomile tea because I love its calming effects.[1]

Chamomile Tea, Brewed

237 grams (8 fluid ounces) 1 cup
236 grams water
2.4 calories
47.4 IU vitamin A
2.4 micromilligrams folate
47.4 milligrams calcium
21.3 milligrams potassium
2.4 milligrams sodium
30.8 micromilligrams fluoride

(*Source:* USDA SR-21 National Nutrient Database for Standard Reference)

While it isn't an intensely flavorful tea (unless you add honey and citrus or it's included in a tea blend), it's an acquired taste. Because of its healing powers for me—both inside and outside the body—I've grown accustomed to drinking it almost every day, in the afternoon and at night. What's more, chamomile tea blends are available. That means vanilla chamomile, green tea and chamomile, and fruit-flavored chamomile herbal teas provide more taste and more health perks.

I'm hardly alone in my love for chamomile tea. Tea master Daniel Johnson's favorite herbal tea is a blend of peppermint and chamomile. "I find the energetics of the floral, sweet, vanilla chamomile and the acrid-dispersing peppermint to be very balanced," he explains. "It is relaxing and clearing," he says, adding, chamomile also "serves as a great foundational tea blend for modification." He further points out that chamomile and mint work together to help soothe the throat and calm the mind. "It is my favorite tea to drink in the evening as an herbal 'nightcap,' which is complemented by a sweet drizzle of local honey." So, the chamomile tea blend Daniel favors relaxes him after a long day, while I turn to it midafternoon and a few hours before bedtime for its relaxation and well-being perks.

In the memorable film *You've Got Mail*, the tea prepared by actor Tom Hanks for Meg Ryan's character may be chamomile. It makes sense because her favorite flower is the daisy, which looks similar to the chamomile flower; and it's comforting while helpful fighting a cold (no doubt due to the stressful event linked to losing her bookstore). In the tea scene, it was a tea bag sitting in a cup served—not strained loose leaves—that caught my eye. I have enjoyed chamomile bag–dunking days and strained loose leaves—both do the trick. But it doesn't end there. . . .

One summer after the hectic Fourth of July holiday that wreaked havoc on my nerves, I tried Evening in Missoula, an herbal blend of chamomile, including raspberry, red clover, rosehips, lemon grass, peppermint, star anise, lavender, and other herbal favorites. At first, I thought: "A basic tea bag of chamomile will do." But after I brewed a cup of the loose leaves of this herbal blend (from The Cozy Tea Cart), I felt I had transcended to a calm place and was glad I took a risk and traveled outside my chamomile comfort zone. And don't forget, I got more of a variety of herbs, so that translates to more healing benefits, too.

Tisane Time: Pour 1 cup of hot water over 1 teaspoon of dried leaves or 1 tea bag. Steep for 4–5 minutes, strain, and add sweet and citrusy orange blossom honey. *Health Check:* Some chamomile brands contain licorice root, which can raise blood pressure. Also, if you are allergic to ragweed, caution is advised. (See more of chamomile benefits in chapter 15, "Home Remedies from Your Kitchen" and chapter 16, "Beau-tea-ful Possibilities.")

CINNAMON (*Cinnamomum zeylanicum*): Not unlike chamomile, cinnamon goes back thousands of years ago, to Egypt and Rome, where cinnamon was used in funeral rites. While calming chamomile is my first tea love, I cannot forget my affair with cinnamon tea, a popular choice I enjoyed in Hollywood, California, back in my early twenties. It was the tea bag paired with a metal tin pot of hot water served with Melba toast at a popular hotel coffee shop on Sunset Boulevard. I use this familiar heart-healthy, immune-boosting, anti-inflammatory herbal tea (loose leaf or finely ground) in baking homemade muffins, tea cakes, candy—and still enjoy a cup of the hot brew. It has a spicy, earthy aroma and flavor that I've missed over the years and drinking it is pleasurable, too. *Tisane Time:* Bring 1 cup of water to boil. Add 1 teaspoon of loose leaf cinnamon. Steep for 10 minutes. Or put 1 tea bag in 1 cup of hot water and steep for 2–3 minutes. Add honey and orange slices to taste. It is also found in tea blends, including chai. (See chapter 5.)

Cinnamon-Cranberry Tea

¼ cup 100% unsweetened cranberry juice
¾ cup purified water
½ teaspoon cinnamon leaves (or to taste) [loose leaves, Harney & Sons]

Combine cranberry juice and water in a small saucepan. Bring to a quick boil. Reduce heat and stir in cinnamon. Serve warm. Serves 1.

(*Courtesy:* Ann Gittleman, Ph.D.)

ECHINACEA (*Echinacea angustifolia*): Another North American perennial I discovered years ago is a favorite herbal tea (especially in the fall and winter months) amongst serious health-conscious food store–goers who want to stave off a serious cold and viruses. Native Americans of the Central Plains turned to echinacea for its immune-boosting properties. Research shows that this herbal tea increases the white blood cells to bolster the immune system. I can personally attest that echinacea is not a great-tasting tea drink. A friend of mine brought me this tea to use after a pesky cold. It ended up in the medicine cabinet and not consumed. *Tisane Time:* Use a tea bag or use 1 teaspoon of loose leaves in a cup of boiling water and steep for 10 minutes. Drink 2 cups a day. Your best bet: Use it with other antioxidant-rich teas (such as white or black tea) with tasty citrus, spices, and honey. *Health Check:* Use echinacea only as soon as you feel a cold or flu coming on—not on a regular basis.

FENNEL (*Foeniculum vulgare*): Fennel is a tisane that you may not be familiar with as an herbal tea but have tasted it in a hearty soup. The Mediterranean herb (it's included in the Oldways Mediterranean Diet) goes back in time to the British herbalist Nicholas Culpeper, who touted the "skinny herb" for its powers to help fight fat. In medieval times, folks believed fennel seeds curbed the appetite. In the 1600s, fennel was known to be a digestive helper. Premenstrual cramps, heartburn, gastrointestinal distress, or want to shed unwanted weight? This herbal drink may be your cup of tea. *Tisane Time:* Put 1 teaspoon loose leaves in 1 cup boiling water. Steep for several minutes. Add honey. Drink as needed.

GINGER (*Zingiber officinale*): Like chamomile and cinnamon, ginger is another favorite of mine and most likely countless other people in the United States and around the globe. It's grown in tropical regions including Asia since ancient times. Versatile ginger was welcomed in the sixteenth century by people from Africa to the Caribbean. Better tasting than echinacea, this herbal tea is touted for its healing virtues and included in many herbal tea blends. Who in the world would eat ginger wrapped in a piece of bread after a big meal to prevent indigestion? As the story goes, ancient Greeks did just that more than four thousand years ago. Gingerroot is known to be a soothing medicine for the stomach, relieving indigestion, premenstrual cramps, and crankies; it can even help you beat cravings because it can calm your nerves and thus inhibit stress eating. *Tisane Time:* Make a decoction by putting 1 teaspoon of gingerroot into 1 cup of boiling water and simmering it for about 10 minutes. Strain and add fresh lemon slices and honey to taste. Or steep a tea bag in 1 cup of boiling water for a few minutes. (Steeping time can be a personal preference based on how strong you like your brew.)

Cold-Fighting Gingerroot Tea

❖ ❖ ❖

1 pint purified water
1 teaspoon fresh gingerroot

Optional ingredients (choose one option):
A pinch of cayenne, 1 large minced garlic clove, and
   the juice of half a lemon (great for when you feel a
   cold coming on)

¾ teaspoon cinnamon (or to taste) or a cinnamon stick
   added upon serving
½ teaspoon ground anise and ½ teaspoon ground
   cloves

   In a small saucepan, fill with water and place gingerroot in it. You can add the optional ingredients. Boil for
about 15–20 minutes. Remove from heat, strain. Add
cinnamon, anise, and cloves for flavor, and enjoy hot or
cold.

(*Courtesy:* Ann Gittleman, Ph.D.)

GINSENG (*Panax quinquefolius*): Rejuvenating ginseng, like ginger,
has been praised for centuries. Its benefits were first noted in a medical book during the Chinese Han dynasty before 100 A.D. It was said
to aid by "quieting the spirit, stopping agitation, and enlightening the
mind." Research shows ginseng, thanks to its ginsenosides, which are
steroid-working compounds, may help boost brainpower, physical energy, and mood, and lessen stress—a culprit that causes havoc on both
the body and brain. *Tisane Time:* Put one tea bag or ½ teaspoon of
loose leaf tea in your teapot. Add ½ teaspoon cinnamon leaves for flavor. Add 1 cup of boiling water and steep for several minutes. Strain,
pour into a mug or cup. Drink only in the morning or early afternoon
since it is a stimulant tea.

LAVENDER (*Lavandula officinalis*): Like chamomile, lavender is another healing herbal tea to use for relaxation. The fabulous aroma is nature's gift. Its roots are located in Europe, Africa, and America where it's gotten a superb reputation in ancient history and the present day for its relaxation powers. This herbal tea can take the edge off anxiety, depression, and headaches. *Tisane Time:* One spring afternoon, out of curiosity I tried brewing lavender loose leaf tea in my coffeemaker. I put 2 teaspoons of the tea into a clean filter. I poured two cups of tap water into the coffee spout. And the amazing scent welcomed me and lingered in the kitchen. I poured a cup and added a bit of honey. It was a sweet, mild herbal tea experience.

LICORICE (*Glycyrrhiza glabra*): Unlike lovely lavender, licorice herbal tea has its own mixed bag of benefits. Native Americans enjoyed licorice tea for its promise of helping a cough to regularity. This versatile herbal tea can also be used for respiratory infections, including cold and flu; it can coat a sore throat, act as an immune booster, and create a sense of calm. *Tisane Time:* As noted I didn't like the flavor of licorice tea when I tasted it for the first time in Eugene, Oregon; I thought it would taste like the black licorice vine candy I chewed as a kid. Your best bet: Blend it with another tea for a better flavor and steep it for less time to avoid bitterness. *Health Check:* Avoid licorice tea if you have high blood pressure, and/or are pregnant or nursing. And remember, licorice root can be an ingredient included in some chamomile teas, so read the ingredients label or contact the manufacturer.

A Loyal Lover of Linden Leaves

Meet Brigitte Almendarez Gavas. She grew up a child of the seventies in a bilingual military family and spent a better part of her childhood between Provence, France, and Naples, Italy. Her exposure to herbal teas is unforgettable. She shares her story and whisks me and now you, too, abroad to her past when a special tisane played a significant role in her life. . . .

There was a tea for everything, constipation, diarrhea, headache, earache, bruises, stomach ache—you name it, I am quite sure I consumed a tea for it. However, the one tea I remember the most is Tilleul (aka linden tea leaves). I did not know for years after my return to the U.S. what the American name for it was. My grandmother suffered from irritable bowel syndrome and the only thing that seemed to comfort her and relieve her digestive pain was a nice hot cup of Tilleul. I remember the subtle floral smell as it was being steeped. To the palate the flower and its beautiful leaves produced a woodsy yet floral taste. One cup of the steeped tea not only relaxed me but would send me into a deep sleep. My mother would give me this tea for not only coughs and colds, but if I was anxious or suffered diarrhea. Once my mom made a paste from the flower to relieve itching from some rash I had acquired. If I was constipated, I was made a tea from the bark . . . yes, the bark of the tilleul tree.

I've tried plenty of other teas, but Tilleul has so many benefits that it is hard to go to other teas. Chamomile is another tea I grew up with. Also a very floral tea, its benefits include relaxing and calming. When raising my children, I gave them chamomile tea rather than Tilleul as it was more difficult to attain here in the U.S. Today, thanks to online stores, I have my stash of Tilleul. I cannot imagine life without tea! I am extremely grateful that my mother and grandmother were able to share their love of teas and their benefits with me.

MARSHMALLOW (*Althaea officinalis*): This herbal remedy like others has been available for centuries. Hippocrates, the father of medicine, used marshmallow to treat wounds. Renaissance herbalists used marshmallow to relieve allergies, sore throats, settle stomach woes, and as a gargle to treat mouth infections. Herbalists believe marshmallow root has a soothing effect on inflammation and sinuses. *Tisane Time:* Use 1 teaspoon marshmallow root in a cup of boiling water. Steep for 10 minutes. Drink a few cups of marshmallow root tea per day until your throat is no longer sore. Wintertime herbal tea blends with marshmallow may include gingerroot and Echinacea.

PEPPERMINT (*Mentha piperita*): Unlike licorice herbal tea, peppermint likely draws more attention because of its taste and it, too, boasts a multitude of perks. Historians say the Romans crowned themselves with peppermint wreaths. Pliny, the Roman scholar, said, "The very smell of it reanimates the spirit." No wonder the colonists brought peppermint to America. Mint tea helped them cope with pesky ailments such as headaches, heartburn, indigestion, and gas. This popular herbal tea is often used for stomach troubles and even menstrual cramps. It's a great way to end a meal—ever notice how restaurants provide mints on the table or by the door?

Peppermint relaxes the muscles of the digestive system, relieving conditions like flatulence and dyspepsia. It also acts as a mild anesthetic to the stomach wall and is useful in treating nausea. It can be used to treat colds, fevers, and flu. Plus, it helps curb anxiety. *Tisane Time:* Steep 1 tea bag or teaspoon of loose leaves in 1 cup of boiling water. Cover and steep for about 5 minutes. Drink a few times daily as needed. It is often used in wellness tea blends. Peppermint bark is one tea that is offered by different tea companies.

RED CLOVER (*Tirifolium pratense*): Not as popular as peppermint tea, red clover does have a following with women. This European weed now grows in North America. It contains good-for-you vitamins, minerals, blood-thinning substances, and plant-based hormones such as isoflavones. According to research, isoflavones may help to stave off hot flashes in menopausal women. Sometimes, hot flashes do not happen until after menopause. If I had used this herbal tea it may have helped me get through the temperature highs and lows after menopause; most likely there are women who can give credit to red clover tea, a ceiling fan, an air conditioner, and layered clothing. *Tisane Time:* Steep 1 bag or 1 teaspoon of dried flowers in 1 cup hot water for several minutes. Best served as iced tea. Add honey to taste.

ROSEMARY (*Rosmarinus officinalis*): Rosemary was known to the Egyptians, and in Rome, where it was used in gardens, it had been linked to love. My first encounter with rosemary is when the herb was used in savory soups and casseroles my mother used to cook. Like other earthy herbal teas, this one brings to the table healing powers, thanks to its flavonoids. Not only is it good for stimulating blood through the heart, it is also good for digestion and relaxation. Proponents claim it is used to stave off allergies. *Tisane Time:* It is also used in a variety of herbal tea blends and pairs well with orange blossom or clover honey.

SAGE (*Salvia officinalis*): This camphor-flavored "fountain of youth" grows wild in the Mediterranean. Its Latin name means "to heal or save." Legend has it that sage will add years to a person's life if used on a regular basis. Sage is believed to cure headaches, hemorrhoids, depression, and other ailments that take a toll on your total health and well-being. *Tisane Time:* Use 1 tea bag or 1 teaspoon dried sage to a cup of boiling water and let steep for 3 to 5 minutes. To improve the slightly medicinal flavor, add honey and lemon to taste. Drink two to three cups daily. *Tisane Time:* Put 1 teaspoon of sage leaves into a cup of hot water. Steep for 3 to 5 minutes, drain. Add honey and a sprig of fresh mint. Sage is used in different herbal tea blends such as parsley and thyme.

Blackberry-Sage Lemonade

❖ ❖ ❖

Put 6½ teaspoons blackberry tea leaves in a natural tea bag with 10 chopped up sage leaves. Pour 3 cups hot water into a large measuring cup and add the tea bag. Steep for 6 minutes (make sure the tea is covered by the water). Pour 3 quarts organic lemonade into a pitcher. Once steeped, strain and remove the blackberry-sage tea bag and pour the tea into the lemonade. Serve chilled. Serves 12–14.

(*Courtesy:* The Cozy Tea Cart.)

FRUIT TEAS

While fruit herbal teas are not my number one favorite, they certainly have their assets, including their lack of caffeine, their richness in antioxidants and vitamin C, and their vibrant colors like red and orange to admire in a glass teacup. These fruity tisanes are kid-friendly. Also, grown-ups get creative and make fruit cocktails or iced fruit tea blends for the spring and summer days, and hot tea wellness blends during the fall and winter months. Blood Orange Fruit Tea and Mango Fruit Tea are two popular varieties, but there is an infinite number of others to attract tea lovers. Brew each one to taste; some people like their fruit tea strong, others like it less potent. Either way, enjoy.

COCONUT (*Cocos nucifera*): Surprise, this is a fruit, not a nut, and it is indeed found in many tea blends. It contains fiber, vitamins, and minerals. Because of its ingredients, it may boost your immunity especially when paired in vitamin C–enriched herbal teas and true healing teas including black tea, white tea, and green tea. It is one of the ingredients in rooibos that adds both memorable flavor and healing perks, ideal for hot tea in colder months but also in the summertime in iced tea.

CRANBERRY (*Vaccinium macrocarpon*): This fruity tea is more exotic than citrus, and fine for autumn and winter seasonal teas. Its pleasant, tart, fruity flavor stems from cranberry bogs. It boasts immune-enhancing vitamin C, dietary fiber, manganese, and flavonoids, such as the heart-enhancing flavonoid rhamnoside. It also contains iron, calcium, vitamins A and B-complex, and some minerals. It is a great fruit tea to use during the cranberry season, such as Thanksgiving and Christmas, and for Valentine's Day infused in a white tea or festive punches (non-alcohol or cocktails) for the summertime. Also, this fruit tea can be used in cooking savory dishes including poultry and lean meat, and sweets (using loose leaves or a strong brew) including cookies, scones, tarts, and breads.

LEMON BALM (*Melissa officinalis*) This flowery, soothing, citrus-flavored herb was named by the Greeks for the bees that buzz around it. It is touted as a "happy herb" because a good night's sleep is good for your spirit. Lemon balm is most often used for anxiety, stress, and insomnia. Lemon balm is often found in a variety of herbal tea blends including different varieties of citrus, but the ones most commonly used for herbal teas are bergamot and dried peeling of orange. Bergamot is used for colds, flu, as well as staving off anxiety, digestive woes, and other respiratory ailments.

ORANGE (*Citrus sinensis*): Another citrusy fruit that is often used in flavored real teas including black tea, white tea, and green tea as well as herbal blends. Like its cousin lemon balm, it is rich in immunity-enhancing vitamin C, fiber, and potassium. It pairs well with a variety of herbal blends including black tea and green tea, too.

POMEGRANATE (*Punica granatum*): Rich in vitamin C, like orange herbal tea, this fruit tea is gaining in popularity. It contains dietary fiber, folate, vitamin K—and polyphenols. While there is no hard-hitting proof this fruit will heal what ails you, its healthy ingredients are nothing to ignore. For New Year's Day I baked a pomegranate ginger cake (for good luck); but it seems easier (removing the seeds from the fruit was a task) and less clean-up (red juice was everywhere) to brew a pot of pomegranate black tea or green tea with pomegranate.

RASPBERRY (*Rubus idaeus*): Like other berry-type teas, this one is rich in vitamin C and can be helpful to bolster your immune system and stave off colds and viruses. This herbal tea is often used in other tea blends including black tea, white tea, and green tea to provide a sweet and tangy note *and* it provides healing powers for wintertime colds and flu, as well as a cooling effect in the summertime.

ROSE HIPS (*Rosa canina*): Rose hips is another notable fruit tea, and a staple in the diets of Native American tribes. Brewing from the berries and incorporating berries in savory dishes were commonplace. Rose hips are a good source of antioxidants including vitamins C, E, and beta carotene, which can help aid the immune system, keeping colds and cough symptoms at bay. Add ½ teaspoon rose hips leaves to black tea (bag or loose leaf) to reap better flavor and better healing benefits. It is often added to different tea type blends.

STRAWBERRY (*Fragaria*): Like rose hips, this is another fruit tisane that is sweet and high in vitamin C and contains some vitamins B and antioxidant E, and minerals. It boasts immune-boosting flavonoids, quercetin and kaempferol, which may help prevent blood platelets from clumping together, and help lower your risk of developing heart disease. It is often included in herbal tea blends for its fruit flavor and aroma. It can make a fine iced tea in the spring or summer, and a delicious winter tea blend with white or green tea.

Wellness Teas Are for What's Ailing Y'All

Wellness teas (tea and herbal blends to help you feel better) are available at supermarkets, health food stores, online, and in luxury health spas. These functional teas serve a purpose—and they are special stand-out brews because they target a specific ailment. California-based Cal-a-Vie Health Spa Signature Teas, for instance, provide their spa-goers with holistic teas, which offer flowers, herbs, and spices grouped by therapeutic benefit. These teas include categories like "Youthful Radiance"—A Skin Care Tea: Antioxidant rich green tea and flower pollen extract (low caffeine) and "Sweet Dreams": calendula, chamomile, catnip, and linden flower, before bedtime (caffeine free).

I can personally attest that the bedtime tea Sweet Dreams took me from my basic cup of chamomile to a better tea place. Not to ignore other groups including "Tummy Tamer," "Cold Cure Organic," "Detoxify Me Organic," and "Mellow Move." It's functional teas like these that attract for a specific purpose and can be beneficial year-round. The choice is up to you, if you prefer to try a prepackaged tea blend or to create your own herbal blends.

These functional teas are sold by companies, but I feel tea is already rich in good-for-you healing ingredients. Actually, I once purchased a lemon wellness tea for a sore throat, but instead of using it, I turned to chamomile and honey, never opening the wellness package. Companies that provide a wellness tea line with catchy titles can and do attract health-conscious folks like me—or someone who has a specific health ailment—but a specialty product may not be needed when a single tea or herbal tea could work just as well.

A cup of basic black tea can be calming, energizing, and helpful to fight off a cold or flu . . . but wellness teas do offer blends that may do the job quicker—or not. I feel if you like the flavor of the brew and it makes you feel better, whether you need an energy boost or calming aid then that's the tea for you. No labels needed. (But note, "Sweet Dreams," the Cal-a-Vie Specialty Tea, converted me to a believer (at least in this one chamomile blend) and allowed me to branch out and be more open to functional teas even though I believe all teas and herbal teas have healing powers.)

THE HEALING POWERS OF HERBAL TEAS AT A GLANCE

These herbal teas can work well alone or can be even more beneficial in herbal blends or in teas (black, white, green, and oolong).

What It Does	Herbal Teas
Anxiety Soothers	Chamomile, Lavender, Linden
Anti-aging Workers	Ginseng, Rooibos, Rosemary, Sage, Gotu Kola
Digestive Helpers	Chamomile, Cinnamon, Ginger, Peppermint
Energizing Aids	Ginseng
Immunity Boosters	Echinacea, Licorice, Marshmallow, Rose Hips
Sleep Inducers	Chamomile, Lavender, Lemon Balm, Passionflower
Stress Relievers	Catnip, Chamomile, Lavender, Linden
Women's Woes	Fennel, Marshmallow Leaf, Raspberry, Red Clover

Ginger Lemon Honey Tea

Just the remedy to pair with homemade fruit scones or muffins, especially if you're feeling a cold or stomach flu paying you a visit, or perhaps the right recipe to keep you healthy if you've been exposed, especially in the fall or winter when germs may pay you an untimely visit. Ginger and lemon go together like salt and pepper—two of nature's finest superfoods with an immunity booster that can keep you healthy.

2 cups water
10 thin slices gingerroot, fresh
1 lemon sliced
3 tablespoons honey (or to taste)
⅓ cup lemon juice

Bring water, gingerroot, and lemon slices to a boil for 1 or 2 minutes. Remove from heat, steep 10 minutes, strain. Stir in honey and lemon juice. Mom would make this tea whenever we came down with a cold. Sometimes she added apple peeling, a piece of onion, and one or two tablespoons of chamomile.

(*Courtesy:* Gemma Sanita Sciabica, *Cooking with California Olive Oil, Treasured Family Recipes*)

Now that I've infused some herbal teas into your brain and daily tea repertoire, in the next chapter you'll find out how teaming teas and tisanes with Mediterranean foods is good for your health and tastes amazing, too.

TEA-CENTRIC HEALING HINTS TO STEEP

✓ Tea types come from the same plant, unlike honey varietals, which come from different plants.

✓ The fruitier the tisane, the more antioxidants and the stronger in flavor and aroma.

✓ Drinking both herbal teas and other teas provides you with different healing powers with their wide range of antioxidants, vitamins, and minerals.

✓ Teas—black, white, green, and oolong—are even tastier and healthier when mixed with herbal teas.

✓ Fruit teas paired with fresh herbs and spices can enhance your immune system, lower your risk of heart disease and cancer, help you to lose unwanted weight, and do much more.

✓ Fruit teas are versatile as a brew during any season or holiday as well as infused in recipes for cooking and baking.

✓ Artisanal herbal teas used in sauces and dressings paired with olive oil, vinegar, honey, chocolate, or coffee add extra flavor and healing powers to superfoods including fish, poultry, salads, and desserts.

PART 5

THE LIQUID OF YOUTH

Tea(s)
Mediterranean-Style

*There is a great deal of poetry and fine sentiment
in a chest of tea.*
—Ralph Waldo Emerson

As an undergraduate student and struggling health journalist, tea helped give me the stamina to liberate dust bunnies and dog hairs for homeowners in the San Francisco Bay Area. My favorite client was a 90-year-old Englishwoman in Nob Hill, a recluse in a fourth-floor apartment overlooking the bay. One overcast morning we shared a pot of ginseng tea and butter cookies. I gave her a bag of plums and lemons from my neighbor's fruit trees. The elderly woman with boundless energy baked a rustic plum tart for us while I vacuumed Oriental rugs and dusted antiques. Once the pastry was baked, we took an elevenses (11:00 A.M. tea break).

Like Kerry Vincent, the Australian judge on Food Network "Challenge" programs who insists on sitting down for a "nice" cup of tea (as English author George Orwell wrote in an essay and British people say and do), my elderly boss served us a hot beverage with milk. It's a time when people relax or problem-solve and while I sipped my tea I spoke. "I won't make my health insurance premium payment this month," I told her but said that I felt invincible—except the scourge of PMS. At the end of the day when she paid me, I noted the check amount was too much. She had covered my insurance. The check was inside an envelope put in a paper bag with two boxes of tea—Earl Grey and lavender. She was another guardian angel who was there for me in time of need as I was for her.

THE MEDITERRANEAN DIET

When I wrote *The Healing Powers of Vinegar*, I was awakened by a fateful meeting with the Mediterranean diet and lifestyle and used it as an underlying theme in the *Healing Powers* series. While I found this timeless diet by accident when researching about red wine vinegar, it made sense to use it as a base, since olive oil is included in the Mediterranean diet and vinegar is paired with oil as well as the superfoods including fruits, vegetables, whole grains, nuts, poultry, and seafood—the diet I'd been following for decades.

True, real teas—black, white, green, and oolong—are *not* on the Oldways Mediterranean Diet Pyramid or food chart, but fruits, herbs, spices, and plenty of water are part of the Oldways Mediterranean Diet Pyramid: a contemporary approach to delicious eating. So once again my superfood of choice—tea—is paired with the diet of choice.

The Mediterranean diet continues to receive praise in the media due to ongoing medical research showing that the diet has healing powers. As the American Heart Association explains it, at least 16 countries border the Mediterranean Sea. Diets, including French, Italian, and Spanish cuisine, differ in the foods of preference but they still include the same food choices in the pyramid.

While I did not go to Europe, as I had noted I would do in the previous *Healing Powers* collection, I did find my way to Montréal, Quebec; Quebec City (French fare is easy to find); and Vancouver, British Columbia (which has both a British and Asian tea influence). Tearooms in these places offer French, English, and Asian-inspired teas and tisanes, ambiance, tea accessories, and cuisine that made me feel like I was visiting abroad in Europe or China instead of a Canadian province. But note, the tea and tisanes environment and the demand for these products play a role in Canada as they do in North America and around the globe.

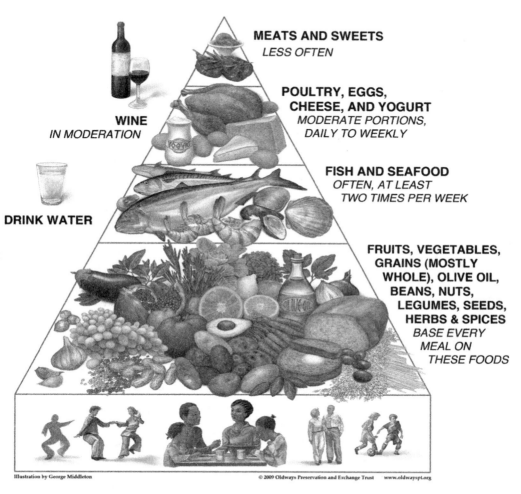

Mediterranean Diet Pyramid
A contemporary approach to delicious, healthy eating

MEATS AND SWEETS
LESS OFTEN

POULTRY, EGGS,
CHEESE, AND YOGURT
MODERATE PORTIONS,
DAILY TO WEEKLY

WINE
IN MODERATION

FISH AND SEAFOOD
OFTEN, AT LEAST
TWO TIMES PER WEEK

DRINK WATER

FRUITS, VEGETABLES,
GRAINS (MOSTLY
WHOLE), OLIVE OIL,
BEANS, NUTS,
LEGUMES, SEEDS,
HERBS & SPICES
BASE EVERY
MEAL ON
THESE FOODS

Illustration by George Middleton   © 2009 Oldways Preservation and Exchange Trust   www.oldwayspt.org

BE PHYSICALLY ACTIVE; ENJOY MEALS WITH OTHERS

A TEA LOVER'S MEDITERRANEAN CLEAN FOODS

In this book, like the other *Healing Powers* series' books, I believe super-foods do contain ingredients that are more powerful when incorporated in the Oldways traditional Mediterranean diet and lifestyle—ranked as one of the top diets in the United States. Some herbs and spices of the Mediterranean diet include lavender, mint, parsley, rosemary, and sage. (Refer to chapter 11, "Healing Herbal Teas".) Here, take a look at my tisane spin on common foods of the Mediterranean Diet Pyramid.

TISANE TREAT #1: Enjoy meatless foods. Eating a plant-based diet, including fruits and vegetables, is healthier and more flavorful if paired with spices and herbs. Also, when serving these foods (such as broccoli, pumpkin, apples, and strawberries) teamed with herbal teas (derived from herbs and spices) they are more appetizing. A *Taste of Herbal Tea:* Cooking and baking with tisanes, and drinking tea paired with eating fruits and vegetables, can make your diet antioxidant-rich(er) and tea-licious.

TISANE TREAT #2: Eat whole green foods. Processed foods (pack-aged eats with ingredients you cannot pronounce) are history, and a trend is to consume whole, fresh food. A *Taste of Herbal Tea:* I include a cup of tea with afternoon tea and an herbal tea before bedtime—and fresh, whole seasonal fruit is often part of the mini-meal.

TISANE TREAT #3: Savor olive oil. I pair extra virgin olive oil with European-style butter infused with sea salt—and I do not use salt often. A *Taste of Herbal Tea:* I often use a wide variety of herb-infused oils *and* herbal teas in cooking and baking. (See chapter 19, "The Joy of Cooking with Tea.")

TISANE TREAT #4: Say hello to saturated fat. High-fat fare has gotten a bad rap for so long but the Mediterranean diet does include saturated fat—about 7 to 8 percent of calories—and 25 to 35 percent of energy. I shun low-fat and non-fat yogurt and cheese because these are often filled with sugar and/or sodium to give the food more flavor as real fat does. A *Taste of Herbal Tea:* Tisanes do not contain fat, sodium, or sugar (unless you put it in your cuppa), so you can use them, like I do, to add pizzazz to foods, in ways such as making glazes and rubs, or in smoothies and real ice cream. Not only will you get the flavor but you'll also enjoy antioxidants, vitamins, and minerals.

TISANE TREAT #5: Cheese and yogurt. Yogurt, including the Greek variety, contains saturated fat but because it is rich in protein and/or calcium, in moderation, no need to stay clear. Goat cheese, crumbled blue cheese, Greek yogurt (I love honey vanilla), organic eggs (brown is my choice), and lean chicken or turkey (on special occasions) are good for you at any age. A *Taste of Herbal Tea:* Enjoying real dairy with spices (such as cinnamon in chai made with organic milk) and herbs (such as mint sprigs in yogurt) and a cup of hot or iced tea (black or white for me, please) is heavenly.

TISANE TREAT #6: Bring on the protein. I am a lacto-vegetarian wannabe-vegan but on occasion I cave and feast on fish (wild salmon or water-packed tuna) and poultry for holiday events (organic chicken and turkey) and a few eggs per week (organic brown ones), including those in baking.

TISANE TREAT #7: Savor sweets. Bring on baklava, biscotti, crème caramel, chocolate, gelato, and fruit tarts! These goodies make you feel good and paired with fresh fruits can be rich in antioxidants. A *Taste of Herbal Tea:* Eating sweets in small portions a few times per week keeps the sweet cravings at bay *and* infused with herbal teas (such as Earl Grey in biscotti or matcha in white chocolate) your sweet tooth will be pampered.

TISANE TREAT #8: Tone down the red meat. Pork and beef are not in my diet but on occasion I will serve them to friends and family. A *Taste of Herbal Tea:* Using an herbal tea rub or marinade with meats can add flavor, aroma, and antioxidants, minerals, and vitamins.

TISANE TREAT #9: Get a move on. The Mediterranean diet includes enjoying an active lifestyle. I swim and walk my dog to achieve that feel-good endorphin "high" (like you get by eating chocolate), to keep both my weight and blood pressure numbers in check, and it helps enhance good sleep. A *Taste of Herbal Tea:* Drinking a cup of hot tea before getting physical and/or after to relax enhances the healing benefits of exercise.

TISANE TREAT #10: Enjoy wine. Wine in moderation is a good thing according to stacks of studies, thanks to its antioxidants from grapes. A *Taste of Herbal Tea:* There is an infinite amount of wine cocktail recipes—combining different wines with herbal tea—that can be delicious and sophisticated, as well as a relaxing beverage (in moderation) for adults.

SIPPING WATER THE MEDITERRANEAN WAY

Drinking plenty of water is part of the Oldways Mediterranean Diet Pyramid. Including water in our daily diet is important for a host of reasons—and getting a portion of it through drinking tea or tisanes is not frowned upon.

I have touted the Mediterranean diet in the *Healing Power* series and it is also an underlying theme in this book due to the herbs, spices, and water. These superfoods are part of a health package; combining these wonder foods will give your meals flavor, and herbal teas made with water will help keep you hydrated—important for good health, well-being, and aging better.

Speaking of age, scientists conducted a study (published in the *Annals of Internal Medicine*) of 10,000 women in their late 50s and early 60s. Fifteen years later, the women who followed the Mediterranean diet, like I do and have been sharing with you in the *Healing Powers* series, stayed healthier as they aged. So a plant-based diet, like you'll find in the Mediterranean diet—paired with herbal teas using herbs, spices, and water—may be the right path to living longer and living better.[1]

TEA-INFUSED EUROPEAN-INSPIRED FOODS

Brewed tea—hot or iced—is everywhere. And it's no surprise to find tea in foods—the kinds that are part of the Mediterranean diet.

Tea Chocolate: Chocolate candy, premium varieties, may contain matcha powdered tea. For instance, white chocolate bars (which can be white or green) combined with Japanese matcha are sophisticated and delicious—perfect for pairing with a cup of tea in the afternoon or after dinner. Japanese Matcha Truffles (like the bars, both from

Mariebelle.com) are soft and rich hand-shaped white chocolate truffles rolled in Japanese matcha tea powder. Also, a box of fine chocolates is fine when infused with spices like cinnamon and cardamom, herbs like lavender and mint, not to forget jasmine—simply tea-licious. A Siam Citron truffle (Vosges Haut) includes jasmine tea, wildflower honey, lemongrass, fresh coconut, white chocolate, and a marigold petal also called calendula. (Refer to chapter 11, "Healing Herbal Teas.")

Tea Cakes: Homemade cakes and cupcakes (I've viewed chefs on Food Network's *Cupcake Wars* show using teas in the baking) can be infused with herbal teas. You can either use ground loose tea leaves or strong brewed tea; cakes combined with lavender or Earl Grey; citrusy herbs like orange and lemon are not uncommon and add sweet, savory, or tangy notes of extra flavor.

Tea Jams: Organic jam is often infused with herbs and spices found in tisanes and is a great way to add flavor to a cup of tea or with fresh scones, muffins, and crumpets.

Tea Honeys: I adore tea-infused honeys like lavender honey crème, lemon, or raspberry honey. Before a radio show, to smooth my voice, I'll put one teaspoon in a cup of chamomile tea—a perfect combination for shaking stage fright. You can make your own by adding herbal leaves of your choice.

Tea-Infused Ice Cream: The first time I tasted tea-infused ice cream was when I purchased Häagen-Dazs Green Tea ice cream. It has a distinct flavor, as does matcha, and it quickly became a common ice cream in my freezer. One half cup contains 250 calories and some vitamin A. It is simple with its ingredients: cream, skim milk, sugar, egg yolk, and green tea. Paired with a tea cookie you've got a sophisticated afternoon snack or fine dinner dessert.

SWEET PICKS: TEA AND DESSERT

Like pairing quality coffee with dessert, your experience with pairing tea can be equally rewarding. But note, there are some tips to help your choice and titillate your palate. And remember, the Mediterranean diet includes desserts, such as fresh fruit, gelato, tarts, and tiramisu, in moderation. So, pick your sweet and tea. (See recipes at the end of each chapter and the last part of this book, "Tea Recipes," for ideas.)

Dessert Pick	Tea
Dark chocolate cakes and cookies. A delicate, fruity dessert; fruit tarts, a dessert containing fresh seasonal fruit	Enjoy a white tea that is light and a bit sweet. White Peony is a perfect pick.
Desserts with a taste of texture such as glazed scones or tea cookies; lemon tarts and pie	Pair them with a grassy green tea or even a nice Jasmine with the mix of green, white, and black.
A rich dessert such as chocolate mousse	A light fruit-flavored white tea or fruity herbal tea can make a sweet balance.
Dark chocolate bark or truffles	A fruit-flavored black tea like cinnamon or lavender with mint is a nice pairing.

MEDITERRANEAN TEAS AND TISANES

In my late twenties, one evening in San Mateo, on the San Francisco Bay Area Peninsula, I was sitting in the kitchen of a male friend from Russia and an older, fatherly Austrian man, a bit like a Wolfgang Puck. He was kindly and offered tea with his homemade bread infused with sunflower seeds and honey. The aroma was inviting and created comfort. Once he took the bread out of the oven and placed it on a cutting board, he brewed a kettle of hot water. My Russian friend sipped a cup of black tea with fresh lemon slices and sugar, while our host took his tea black with sugar cubes. I was served a cup of hot water and added my own chamomile tea bag, plain. One by one, we cut slices of warm bread slices topped with pats of real butter. During tea time, our words were heartfelt, dishing about life's ups and downs in Europe and America: loss of lovers, family members, job changes, and money challenges. It was tea that gave us incentive to share mindfulness, compassion, laughter, and ideas. That night's dangling conversation still lingers in my mind decades later despite our different backgrounds and tea tastes—we shared tea and sympathy.

Tea cultures vary throughout the United States—sweet tea in the South to herbal tea in the Pacific Northwest and around the world. When I visit different states and countries, it is fascinating how the tea types differ. In my home state of California (a melting pot of Mediterranean culture but with West Coast roots), green, black (flavored types), and herbal teas are popular in supermarkets, coffee shops, homes, and colleges. In the Pacific Northwest it seems like herbal teas (especially fruit varieties in Seattle, Washington) are popular and offered in restaurants and luxury hotels. But tearooms offer a wide range of teas and tisanes.

When I was in flight to the East Coast and laid over in Georgia, iced tea—ready to drink (an array of flavors) and the standard beverage at restaurants was easy to find. After all, it's a refreshing treat when the temperature is higher than 80 degrees and iced tea is welcome for visitors and locals of all ages.

In the eastern province of Quebec, a place of European people and French cuisine, herbal teas including chamomile, linden, and mint are not difficult to find, whether it be in hotel rooms, bistros in Quebec City (or on the train en route to it), or in the airport. Italian restaurants that I've frequented in the San Francisco Bay Area (a city that is diverse like Montréal) offer classic black tea; and I've heard that herbal teas, like my favorite, chamomile, are offered to people (especially if feeling a bit under the weather) in Italy. Remember, as I noted earlier, it is the place where Brigitte grew up and enjoyed linden herbal tea, used especially to stave off a cold or flu.

When I visited the West Coast province of British Columbia, I noticed an Asian influence at hotels and tearooms. So it was no surprise a variety of tea including black, green, oolong, white, and specialty teas were offered. And tea masters who have traveled to Asian countries share tales of drinking green tea paired with Asian cuisine.

While I'm not familiar with Indian food (although my mother used to make curry powder dishes that I didn't eat), I do know cultivation of tea is India's second largest industry following tourism. When I entertained an Indian photograph crew for a book I penned on earthquakes, I did serve coffee. If I could have a redo, I'd brew a pot (or two) of chai (loose leaf) with all the wonderful spices, use soy milk, and offer honey to sweeten the pot.

All of these places and teas available can appeal to tea lovers. Also, it is believed that it's not just tea that helps people keep their weight in check—people who incorporate tea into their diet often engage in a healthier lifestyle that includes eating a good diet and exercising regularly. But that's not to say a tea-infused diet can't help you to lose weight and keep it off. It can.

In the next chapter, you'll find out that tea is a super fat fighter. The best part is, once you enter the world of tea the choices will woo you and drinking tea will be a wonderful way to help you get and stay lean, thanks to its amazing ingredients that I'll tell you about so you can enjoy tea even more.

Pretty Plum Earl Grey–Infused Tart

This is my own recipe inspired by growing up in San Jose, California—a place once teeming with plum orchards. I remember as a kid, when walking to different swimming pools during the summer months, picking plums off trees in orchards was a normal thing to do. But nowadays, San Jose is citified, so this tart takes me back in time when life had a slower pace, was simpler, and fruit desserts could be homemade by getting fruit from the neighborhoods.

1 store-bought premium pie crust or make your own
    from scratch
5 plums (firm like apples work best), sliced in wedges
    (with skins left on)
8 tablespoons granulated white sugar
1 teaspoon lemon rind
2 teaspoons lavender tea, loose leaf, finely ground
1/8 cup organic strawberry preserves, melted
Confectioners' sugar
Walnuts, finely chopped (optional)
Fresh mint sprigs for garnish

Line a rectangular pan with parchment paper. Unroll refrigerated single pie crust. Simply shape into a rectangle (it is very easy to do this). Fold edges so they are thick but not perfect to give your tart a rustic, European look (like you would find in a bistro in Italy). Fill with plum slices (cut in the same size) in rows and layer. Sprinkle with sugar, lemon rind, and tea. Bake at 350 degrees for 40 to 50 minutes till crust is golden and fruit is bubbly. Remove and spread top with preserves. Sprinkle with sugar and top with nuts. Cool. Place in fridge to set. Slice in nice-sized rectangles. Serves 8.

A plum tart, like this one, is vibrant in color. Because the store-bought pie crust comes with two rolls, you make another fruit tart (apple or pear pairs well with Earl Grey tea and lemon). I savored the plum treat at night on the deck under the big, bright full moon. It took me back to the charm of San Francisco. Each bite of tart was like enjoying the exciting city lights and calming majestic mountains. Teamed with a cup of white tea, it is heavenly.

TEA-CENTRIC HEALING HINTS TO STEEP

✓ The Oldways Mediterranean Diet Pyramid and food chart includes herbs, spices, and water—components of herbal tea.
✓ The Mediterranean diet and lifestyle is used around the world and you can enjoy it wherever you are—including regular exercise with drinking plenty of water to stay hydrated.
✓ On the road, drinking plenty of water and herbs (included in herbal teas) and Mediterranean common foods (including fruits, vegetables, and whole grains) were my staples.
✓ The Mediterranean Diet and Lifestyle Pyramid, according to studies, may help lower the risk of developing heart disease, cancer, and obesity.

The Skinny on Tea and Fat

Love and scandal are the best sweeteners of tea.
—Henry Fielding, *Love in Several Masques*, IV, xi

During the summer before attending graduate school, I pulled *The Graduate* classic film act, my way. Evicted from a San Jose garden apartment (dogs were no longer allowed), Stone Fox, my canine sidekick Labrador retriever, and I traveled to the Gold Country of California, and camped at Tuolumne River.

On a warm morning, a motor boat full of middle-aged vacationers docked their craft at the riverbank below our modest campsite. Two couples left an ice chest on a blanket, and sped off water-skiing. Like two coyotes, my hungry companion and I scurried down the hill. I opened the chest; Stoney retrieved a package of cold cuts. I seized a bag of ice and a jar of instant tea and fruit; and stuffed the food in my backpack. Running up the slope back to our site was a Bonnie and Canine feat. The reward: Meat and water for my pooch—lemon-flavored tea and fresh fruit for me. Hours later the boaters searched the riverbank for their MIA stuff. I waved, my dog barked. It was survival of the fittest (with a nod to Herbert Spencer, who discovered the theory of struggling to survive) and tea (a special thanks to Nestle USA, who debuted instant tea back in 1946) made those lean, summertime days bearable.

Each time you lift a teacup to your eyes, nose, and lips, as I did that summer, you have a perfect way to relax—and a natural remedy to help you lose unwanted pounds. Tea time, morning, afternoon, and night, can give you the chance to find your balance and is a dieter's best friend. Nutritionists at health spas will tell you that they serve tea because it can help drinkers to feel a sense of peace. Drinking tea is not a trend, it is a way of life that goes back centuries—and it often is teamed with a healthy lifestyle.

SIPPING TEA CAN HELP YOU LOSE WEIGHT

Top experts, including Dr. Mehmet Oz, confirm a cup of tea (different types that he dished on his TV program *The Dr. Oz Show*) may boost body fat loss. According to diet gurus and studies, mounting evidence shows how compounds in tea and tisanes—this healthy, functional superfood—can work as a dieter's aid to lose both unwanted fat and pounds.

Past research proves the caffeine in tea can up your calorie-burning power for a few hours after drinking a cup. Also, it's believed by medical doctors that the polyphenols in tea—such as black tea, white tea, and green tea—can help reduce belly fat. Evidently, its antioxidants (catechins), when paired with caffeine, can boost your metabolism, which can end up in weight loss, according to past research. And that's not all . . .

There are also other fat-fighting perks experienced by women, like me, perhaps, you, too: less hunger, staying regular (this can reduce bloat and feeling sluggish, which too often can keep you from exercising), and a boost in energy. "Black tea provides a comforting beverage with many positive health benefits. It can fill you up for a minimal calorie impact (unless you add sweeteners)," points out dietitian Vandana Sheth, adding that this type of tea also "provides a quick pick-me-up from the caffeine."

A revitalizing aid like caffeine (in moderation because too much can trigger stress eating) can help you stay within a healthful calorie intake per day as well as give you energy to get moving—enabling you to build muscle mass, which burns calories and is key to staying lean and fit.

Less is more when adding sugar to your daily tea or diet. The American Heart Association recommends no more added sugar per day than 9 teaspoons for men, 6 teaspoons for women. So, as an alternative option, the natural flavor and notes of tea and tisanes (especially fruit and spice herbal teas) can feed your sweet tooth and help curb cravings to overindulge in high-fat or sugary treats with empty calories. Sheth shares that she enjoys drinking chai with milk and spices. "It brings back wonderful memories of growing up in India," she recalls. Earl Grey's flavor and fragrance reminds her of high tea and her go-to brews for warmth and comfort on cool days are peppermint or green tea.

And it gets even better because herbal teas help lower stress, which can wreak havoc on the body and often lead to overindulging in comfort food that is full of sugar and fat, which can pack on pounds and body fat. Also, stress can increase the hormone cortisol, which is believed to pack on belly fat.

DRINK MORE TEA, LOSE MORE GIRTH

Water may be a dieter's best friend—and tea is not excluded. Here's proof: Health professor Ruopeng An of the University of Illinois and researchers have pinpointed by increasing your water intake by one to three cups per day you may eat 68 to 2,015 fewer calories on a daily regimen. The eye-opening study published in the *Journal of Human Nutrition and Dietetics* included more than 18,000 people who not only experienced a decrease in calories, but ate less fat, sugar, and sodium and cholesterol foods. The result? Fewer calories, more weight loss.

What's more, good news for tea lovers (especially if drinking water isn't your cup of tea) because beverages such as unsweetened black tea and herbal tea were not included as sources of plain water, but their water content was included in the calculations of the individuals' water intake. It was noted that decreases were more among men and among young and middle-aged adults, who may be likely to eat more calories per day.[1]

And remember, drinking water plays a role in the Oldways Mediterranean Diet Pyramid and guidelines.

A TOAST TO SKINNY TISANES

So drinking more water and teas can help you to get and stay leaner at any age but there are some herbal teas that may help you to lose unwanted body fat and pounds a bit faster and more easily. Herbs that can help stimulate water loss are called herbal diuretics. They include dandelion, marshmallow root, parsley, and uva ursi. Some of these herbal teas are used solo or in tea blends by spa-goers for their dieting benefits without feeling like you're dieting.

Some nutritionists have explained that herbs like these can help you feel slimmer because they aid in losing water weight and hydrate you, which can give your skin a wonderful glow. And yes, I've experienced these rewards by turning to a few of these reducing teas, especially during hormonal changes from premenstrual syndrome (PMS), perimenopause, menopause—and even post-menopause. I can personally attest that herbal diuretics help get rid of water retention, aka bloat. Here, take a look at a few of my past and present favorite tried-and-true tisanes that may be your cup of tea.

DANDELION (*Taraxacum officinale*): Meet a skinny herbal tea that is popular because it is a good aid if you're eating less and losing more weight. Dandelion is rich in potassium, much like water-dense fresh fruits and vegetables. This, in turn, makes the herb a diuretic, which means you get rid of excess water weight—the culprit that can make you look and feel bloated. Dandelion also contains some minerals including calcium, iron, and vitamin A—all wanted when you are budgeting calories. Dandelion root is available at health food stores, specialty tea shops, and online. Put 1 teaspoon of dandelion root in a cup of hot water. Steep for several minutes, and add a bit of honey (it can help provide energy to burn calories and is only 21 calories per 1 teaspoon).

PARSLEY (*Petroselinum crispum*): Parsley is better known by people but dandelion is an up-and-coming herbal tea in the dieter's world. Like dandelion, parsley contains good-for-you nutrients—it's not just a garnish. Most important, it has pound-paring benefits because of its diuretic effect—it can help you to dump water weight, a godsend for women during hormonal shifts. Follow the same brewing method as dandelion. Opt for fresh parsley. Add a squeeze of fresh orange, lime, or lemon to make it tasty. (*Health Check:* Not advised for pregnant women.)

Lose Up to 7 Pounds on the 3-Day Vacation Weekend Tea Mini-Fast

Mini-Fast

Here is a jump-start diet plan. It is not intended to be used long-term. But you can use it one day per week or as needed after the first time, since it gives your body a vacation from overindulging in holiday food, special occasions serving rich, high-calorie fare. Eating clean foods from a plant-based diet (including nature's berries, nuts, and seeds that'll fill you) will help give your body a break—detoxing from sugar, meat, dairy, bad fats, refined carbs, and processed foods. Plus, it can help you to lose unwanted pounds (which can increase as you age because you lose more muscle mass). Taking a mini-fast food vacation can help you get fit and dump the muffin top, too.

This diet plan is an adaption from umpteen mini-fasts I've created with the help of nutritionists. It also uses foods in the Oldways Mediterranean Diet Pyramid. Most important, it's one I've tried and know firsthand that it works.

The Rules

- Do not go below 1,000 calories. Keep in mind, olive oil contains 120 calories per tablespoon.
- Do not eat after 7 P.M. If you are hungry, you may eat a piece of fresh fruit with herbal tea.
- If preferred, you may substitute protein choices with tofu, eggs, beans, or brown rice. Fruit choices can be changed as long as it is fresh.
- Health authorities advise you to drink 6–8 8-ounce glasses of water daily. The amount depends on your size and weight, activity level, and where you live; seasons count, too (you may require more in a hotter climate).

- Consume 1 cup of black and/or white tea (1–2 times per day—hot or iced).
- Drink herbal tea (any kind). You may replace one or two glasses of water with tisanes.
- Consult with your health practitioner before starting this diet, a new tea or herbal tea, or any new diet plan. Do not use if you're pregnant, nursing, or have diabetes.
- Take a daily multivitamin to help you get adequate nutrients.

Breakfast:

Berries (no limit but moderation is best)
Coffee or tea (1 cup black or white)
Snack
Herbal tea

Lunch:

4 oz. fresh white turkey meat or chicken breast
Salad greens with olive oil, vinegar (your choice—apple cider or red wine), and spices/herbs to taste
Tea (1 cup black or white)

Snack:

Herbal tea

Dinner:

6–8 oz. flounder, salmon, or sole
Green vegetable (your choice) with fresh lemon (suggestions: artichoke, asparagus, spinach)
1 cup fresh berries

Snack:

Herbal tea
Snacks
Fresh fruit (apple, orange, pear)
Raw vegetables (carrots, celery)

BABY BOOMER BRIGITTE LOST 10 POUNDS!

A health-conscious woman, Brigitte Almendarez Gavas in Dover, Delaware, was inspired to try the no-frills Tea Mini-Fast. "I've been putting off formally trying to lose weight. I don't believe in dieting, as I believe if I eat healthy and exercise, I can maintain a healthy life." But her doctor advised the busy boomer to shed some pounds, especially since she had been coping with arthritis. So, Brigitte, who tagged herself as "fit fat," took the Tea Mini-Fast challenge—and used Northeastern cuisine with a European twist. "I felt full all day, therefore I had more energy from Day 1. The struggle was giving up my dark chocolate before bed." As the days passed, "the fruit, water, and tea filled me up" and her friends and family told her she was "glowing." Four pounds lighter in three days, she said, "I'm looking forward to more weight loss."

Day 1

32 ounces water (Evian) throughout the day

Pre-breakfast:
6 ounces warm water with lemon

Breakfast:
8 ounces coffee
1 bowl fresh strawberries (local)
1 cup herbal tea (chamomile apricot)

Lunch:
1 salad: Combine kale and spinach, 1 tablespoon sunflower seeds, strawberries, cranberries in moderation, 3 ounces tunafish, drained, 1 tablespoon olive oil mixed with balsamic vinegar to taste
2 small apricots
1 cup iced green tea with mint, cucumber, lemon

Snack:
1 handful almonds, 3 dates
1 cup hot green tea

Dinner:

 3 ounces salmon, grilled in marinated lemon juice, with oregano and rosemary, ½ cup brown rice (organic) with sautéed sweet pepper and onions, 1 small side dish of salad greens topped with sunflower seeds, drizzled with 1 tablespoon olive oil and a splash of balsamic vinegar

---

Day 2

Pre-breakfast:

 6 ounces warm water with lemon

Breakfast:

 8-ounce cup of coffee
 1 bowl of fresh strawberries
 1 cup herbal tea (chamomile apricot)

Lunch:

 1 salad: Combine kale and spinach, 1 tablespoon sunflower seeds, watermelon chunks, strawberries, cranberries in moderation, 3 ounces tunafish, drained, 1 tablespoon olive oil mixed with balsamic vinegar to taste
 1 banana
 1 cup iced green tea with mint, cucumber, and lemon

Snack:

 1 handful almonds, 3 dates
 1 cup hot green tea

Dinner:

 3 ounces grilled swordfish marinated in lemon juice, oregano, and rosemary
 ½ cup brown rice (organic) with sautéed zucchini and eggplant
 1 small side salad greens and seeds with 1 tablespoon olive oil and balsamic vinegar to taste

Day 3

Pre-breakfast:
6 ounces warm water with lemon

Breakfast:
Fruit Smoothie: 1 cup mix of watermelon, strawberries, pineapple and 1 cup coconut milk

Snack:
Herbal tea (iced linden tea, watermelon slices, and mint)

Lunch:
1 salad: Combine kale and spinach, 1 tablespoon pecans, mandarins, cranberries in moderation, 3 ounces chicken (white meat), 1 tablespoon olive oil mixed with apple cider vinegar to taste
1 cup iced green tea with mint, cucumber, and lemon

Snack:
1 handful almonds, 3 dates
1 cup iced green tea with mint, cucumber, lemon

Dinner:
3 ounces grilled salmon marinated in lemon juice, oregano, and rosemary
½ cup brown rice (organic) with sautéed sweet peppers and sweet onions
1 small side salad greens with 1 tablespoon olive oil and balsamic vinegar to taste
Brigitte's Top Tips: In the morning include yoga and meditation, and in the afternoon swim and/or engage in aqua therapy. "You'll be energized and feel healthier!"

Fruit Compote with Spice Tea and Walnuts

Fruit compote goes way back in time. This black tea–based fresh fruit recipe provides a sweet and spicy twist with spice tea, not to ignore the nuts. It's a sophisticated dessert to serve up for autumn or winter—a delight. To enhance this healing foods treat, pairing it with an earthy black tea (may I suggest a flavored black tea with vanilla) will make it a sweet pleasure to love.

2–3 apples
2–3 pears
2 tablespoons spice tea (or black tea with clove,
     orange peel, or cinnamon)
⅓ cup water
2 tablespoons maple syrup
½ cup raisins
1½ tablespoons organic lemon juice
Cinnamon, to taste
1 cup walnuts, chopped

Wash, core, and chop apples and pears into slices or chunks. Place in large saucepan with tea and water. Add maple syrup and raisins. Cook over medium heat, stirring occasionally, for 10 minutes. Add lemon juice and cinnamon. Cook for another 10 minutes, until soft. Top warm fruit with nuts and enjoy. Serves 4.

(*Courtesy:* The Cozy Tea Cart)

Speaking of tea and tarts, in the next chapter, you'll learn that living in the world of tea you may turn the clock back. The wide range of anti-aging teas and tisanes are amazing—and are part of the superfoods parade that will help you stay healthy, maintain your weight, stall age-related diseases, and live a longer, happier life.

TEA-CENTRIC HEALING HINTS TO STEEP

✓ Tea-infused desserts (homemade or store-bought) are becoming more popular, are better for your health, and in moderation can curb your sweet tooth so you don't overindulge.

✓ Drinking a flavored black tea (such as caramel) can fill your craving for a caramel dessert and you won't consume unwanted calories, fat, or sugar.

✓ Green tea with caffeine and the compound EGCG boost calorie-burning power, past research reveals.

✓ The French Paradox makes sense. French people who do eat mini meals with fresh fruits, herbs, and spices stoke their calorie-burning power so they lose weight easier.

✓ Eating healthy fats like olive oil and fatty fish provides satiety so you won't be tempted to overeat.

✓ Herbal teas can help you lose unwanted pounds, water weight, and bloat.

✓ Both tea and fruits have been found to contain antioxidants—a myriad of compounds that are linked to heart health, lowering the risk of developing cancers, and boosting longevity.

✓ Pairing the right tea with the right desserts is an art that can be learned for your palate and health's sake.

Age-Defying Dream Potion

*Surely a pretty woman never looks prettier
than when making tea.*
—Mary Elizabeth Braddon, *Lady Audley's Secret*

After completing graduate school (the brainpower-boosting ingredients in tea did help me study and pull a few all-nighters), I fell into the world of writer for hire. Once again, I relied on tea and its energizing benefits, as I was often juggling deadlines as a health journalist. Drinking black tea (hot or iced depending on the season) kept me going physically and mentally. But tea and tisanes were there for me during seasonal and big life changes like in the classic Byrds' song "Turn! Turn! Turn!"

My dad, at 74, was diagnosed with cancer. My sibling and I visited him at the hospital and I recall one sobering night. I brought photos of him and his Navy crew; at our favorite swimming pool; training the Dalmatian, Casey, he gave to me. I had a dream that night of my dad, remembering a fun-loving man who took me, a teen, to San Jose Municipal Airport one summer night. We drank Arnold Palmers—a non-alcoholic sweet tea–lemonade drink created by the professional golfer—and stood outside on the lookout tower and watched airplanes soar into the sky. He passed at noon the next day. I brewed a pot of tea like the character Patrick Jane of TV's *The Mentalist,* a tea addict who faces death in his job and his words ring true: "Tea? It's like a hug in a cup." I agree.

STALL FATHER TIME

Tea and sympathy are a pair that goes back centuries—as does searching for the fountain of youth. While baby boomers and anti-aging medical doctors in the 21st century attempt to stall the aging process, tea is one superfood that is on the age-defying list. Pick your teas and tisanes paired with Mediterranean diet foods to turn back the hands of time—and you may add years to your life, reveal medical researchers.

Studies show that when you eat a variety of antioxidant-rich functional foods, including tea, your chronological age will increase, and your biological age will decrease, meaning your body age may be lower and that, in turn, means you may be able to live a longer, higher-quality type of life.

No matter what stage you are in your life, tea can be helpful. As the graying of America is happening, tea can be your best friend no matter what generation you are in because it may enhance your health and well-being as you grow older. The healthier you are, the younger your body stays. While we all have expiration dates (and most of us have lost loved ones to age-related diseases), you may be able to increase your "shelf life" if you take care of yourself and that includes drinking tea.

Here are some age-defying strategies that remind me of the characters' in the classic *The Wizard of Oz,* who search for their personal best, be it by way of a brain, courage, heart, or ultimate happiness . . . all things you may find through tea.

BRAIN. Age-related neurological challenges in memory and cognition happen, but medical researchers are discovering that diet—including tea—may help stall or even prevent brainpower issues. The benefits of tea that help improved biomarkers for reducing risk of heart disease may improve brain health, too. The antioxidants in tea may be one avenue to help protect brain cells from the scourge of free radicals. Past studies show that green tea's catechins, theanine, and eipigallocatechin-3 gallate (EGCG), may be the good guys that keep our brain working as it should and the way we want it to function.

Also, past research (but not human studies) show the promise of both green and black tea thanks to theanine (a brain-enhancing amino acid) that might be the link to guarding against Alzheimer's disease—something that affected my beloved Brittany, Simon, at the age of 12½—weeks after I had viewed the award-winning film *Still Alice* while sipping tea in my hotel room in Vancouver, British Columbia. It was a sign to me that neurological decline can affect anyone.

BONES. While caffeine has been said to be a risk factor for brittle bones or osteoporosis, those who drink tea have been found to have higher bone mineral density. Drinking tea has also been shown to boost bone-building markers and improve muscle mass—both of which may lower the risk for broken bones and fractures.

Scientists have found that polyphenols in green tea may help improve bone quality and strength. Drinking tea was linked with a 30 percent reduced risk in hip fractures among men and women 50 years of age or older.[1]

Incorporating white tea in your diet repertoire may help you also lessen your risk of rheumatoid arthritis, according to researchers at Kingston University in London. Scientists put to test more than 20 plant and herb extracts. The findings: The plants had healing benefits, but white tea was the superstar with its age-defying antioxidants, which may show that white tea lessens the risk of inflammation, a trait of arthritis.[2]

HEART. The American Heart Association says that folks who drink 1–3 cups of tea a day have a lower risk of heart failure than those who never drank tea, according to a study presented at the American Heart Association's Epidemiology/Lifestyle Scientific Sessions.[3]

TEA TIME AT ANY AGE

In Your 20s: At 20-something, you're at your physical best—sometimes. People at this age, if in good health thanks to genes and lifestyle choices, believe they're invincible. Often, they do not even get health insurance because they feel they will not need it. Despite taking a gamble with or without insurance, drinking tea on a daily basis is insurance in its own way.

Black, white, and green tea are ideal choices for this age group. The age-proofing antioxidants will lay the groundwork for a healthy heart. Also, the caffeine in black tea, especially, will help provide the incentive to exercise—a key to getting and staying lean and fit.

In Your 30s: In your 30s, like your 20s, your mind and body are often in good shape if your diet, exercise program, and lifestyle choices are good ones. Get annual checkups, including a dental checkup twice a year; tea is acidic, which may cause problems for some people's teeth. (See chapter 18 for tips on having your tea and drinking it too.)

White and green tea are good selections for this age group. Both teas contain caffeine, but as noted earlier, less than black tea, but enough to give you the extra energy for both your mind and body. Also, adding a few tisanes—such as rooibos and chamomile—to stay balanced and enhance your immune system with its antioxidants is a smart choice.

In Your 40s: In your 40s, women and men enter middle age. During these years chronic health issues can occur, including weight gain, changes in normal numbers for blood sugar, cholesterol, and blood pressure.

Black, white, and green tea are excellent choices—and mixing them up to get all the benefits is an excellent idea. You don't want to drink too much black tea all day long because the caffeine could increase anxiety or blood pressure. But a cup in the morning or afternoon could help give you the energy to exercise, boost mood, and lessen stress—all good things.

In Your 50s: Welcome to the years when medical checkups may include tests to ensure you stay healthy and prevent diseases—from heart disease to type 2 diabetes. The upside is, if you have been drinking tea in the past decades and continue to do so, you may not face these health challenges. Like in your 40s, including a mix of teas is a good idea but adding more tisanes (such as immune boosters and heart helpers) can help you get through the midlife changes and move on into the next passage.

In Your 60s-Plus: During this decade and throughout the golden years people often must face health ailments including diseases that are genetic; but you can avoid lifestyle-related illnesses by making healthier changes. Many of these obstacles can be prevented or stalled with the help of diet, exercise—and teas and tisanes. Black, white, and green teas are excellent choices in moderation—both drinking and incorporating them in foods. But natural tisanes for the immune system, heart health, energy, and getting good sleep are godsends from nature.

LONGEVITY-BOOSTING TEAS THROUGHOUT YOUR LIFETIME

Tea Type	Disease-Fighting Healing Powers	Some Anti-aging Nutrients
Black	Cancer, heart disease	Antioxidants, caffeine
(Dark, Pu'er)	Digestion	Probiotics
White	Cancer, diabetes, heart disease	Polyphenols
Green	Cancer, immune system, heart health	Flavonoids, catechins, vitamin C, EGCG
Oolong	Cancer, heart disease	Antioxidants, caffeine
Herbal	Depression, low energy	L-theanine
Rooibos	Asthma, immune system	Aspalathin and nothofagi

Green and Cran-Orange Tea

This recipe is adapted from a health spa tea recipe I've used, but I gave it a new spin. The healing foods from Mother Nature are not only good for you but they also taste superb, sweet and tart. You can use this brew year-round, hot or iced, and it's also a wonderful detox tea (great for post-holidays and overindulging or in the springtime), thanks to the cranberry juice.

2 cups water
1 cup cranberry juice, organic
½ cup orange juice, organic
2 green tea bags
1 tablespoon honey
2 orange slices for garnish

Combine water and both cranberry and orange juices in a medium-size pot set over medium heat. Bring to a simmer. Place the green tea bags into a warmed teapot, pour in the hot cran-orange-water mixture. Add honey. Steep for 3 minutes. Pour into teacups. Garnish with orange slices. Serves 3.

Speaking of tea and good health, in Part 6, "Tea Cures," you'll get a taste of how honey and how teaming different types of tea and tisanes are the natural path to tending to annoying and chronic health ailments, including allergies, colds, sore throats, and so much more.

TEA-CENTRIC HEALING HINTS TO STEEP

✓ Medical doctors and scientists are now confirming what herbalists have known for years—tea has a variety of healing powers.
✓ Throughout history, ancient cultures have used tea to stay healthy and live longer.
✓ Antioxidant-rich "real" teas, including black, green, oolong, and red, paired with darker honeys provide extra healing properties.

PART 6

TEA CURES

Home Remedies from Your Kitchen

I am so fond of tea, I could write a whole dissertation on its virtues.
—James Boswell, *Boswell's London Journal*

After living one fourth of my life in a San Francisco Bay Area European-style historic upstairs bungalow with a stunning view of the San Carlos hills (with memories of admiring the fog at dawn and with the city light) while sipping a cup of steaming black tea in the mornings and iced herbal teas at night), my peninsula days were history. I moved to Lake Tahoe but my love for tea did not die.

In fact, my love for traveling across America and Canada blossomed. I booked a flight to Montréal, Quebec—a place I hitchhiked to in my twenties and fled when I discovered it was French-speaking, and the fast past scared me. I vowed to return when I became an author.

Decades later I found myself getting up at 2:30 A.M. to catch a 6:00 A.M. plane to Salt Lake City, then to Atlanta, Georgia, to Montréal. Waking up without adequate sleep felt odd and it was the wrong hour to brew coffee. So, I made a cup of my own blend: black and green tea. It gave me energy enough to get on the shuttle bus without acting like a zombie from a sci-fi film.

But while tea offers home cures, including beating sleepiness, it can also keep you calmer than java. It turns out when I was in the TSA line I was asked by the agent: "Have you ever been searched?" I answered: "No," and calmly I was led into a booth and patted down. I was told it was the metal on my boots and layered clothing that got me into this uncomfortable position. I was thankful for the tea because coffee might have made me combative or sarcastic. I had the right complacent attitude and made it into the waiting room for the flight. At a counter café, I ordered a cup of hot water and used my own chamomile tea bag to keep me calm enough for the next fear factor: flying out of the Sierra and into Salt Lake City—two airports known for turbulent flights.

I'll describe 50 common health ailments from A to Z and provide why there is a growing trend of at-home tea cures, including black, white, green, and red (and some non-tea tisanes not already discussed) that'll wow you with their potential healing powers. I sprinkled in tea wisdom from tried-and-true folk remedies, scientific studies, medical experts, and my own home tea and tisane cures.

Steeping Guidelines for a Perfect Cuppa

For white, green, and oolong teas use very hot water and steep for 2–3 minutes. Black teas use very hot water to a full boil and steep for approximately 3 minutes. When brewing herbal teas, use very hot to a full boil and steep about 5 minutes. The time of steeping can vary and be your preference—whether you like a brew light or strong. But note, a good guide to follow is that green, white, and oolong take less time to steep, black a bit longer, and herbals even longer. Also, for best results, use the instructions (which can vary) of the individual tea brand often on the box or tea tin.

1 **ALLERGIES (Stop the sneezing.)** Are you sneezing, coughing, and rubbing your watery eyes? Sounds like you're one of millions of allergy sufferers, and it's worse during springtime and fall when

pollen soars and other allergens, including dust mites, dust, and pet dander can wreak havoc on your immune system.

What Tea Rx to Use: Opt for 1 or 2 cups of green or white tea (hot or iced) mixed with mild honey.

Why You'll Feel Tea-rrific: Taking over-the-counter allergy medications can work but they often come with side effects, such as dry mouth, anxiety, and even lightheadedness. With green tea or white tea (rich in anti-inflammatory and immune-boosting antioxidant quercetins), you can be on your way to beating symptoms from allergens. A bonus: Tea is less expensive than taking allergy medication, especially if you resort to prescription meds or even shots by an allergist. Try tea and honey to fight those allergens.

2 **ANEMIA (Boost your energy.)** Coping with allergens is a pesky problem and often seasonal, but facing a lack of dietary iron comes with a mixed bag of obstacles, too. In my late teens, I was diagnosed with borderline anemia. Blame it on fad weight loss diets, and not getting adequate iron-rich foods. Anemia can give you telltale signs, including feeling lightheaded, bleeding gums, and fatigue. But tisanes can help boost your iron intake and come to the rescue.

What Tea Rx to Use: Heat 1 cup of water and add 1 heaping teaspoon of red raspberry leaf or dandelion herbal tea. Steep for 4–6 minutes. Repeat 2 times per day. Incorporate iron-rich foods into a healthful Mediterranean diet, including poultry, seafood, apricots, spinach, and fortified whole grain cereals.

Why You'll Feel Tea-rrific: By sipping a hot cup of herbal tea paired with foods rich in iron, you can keep your weight in check and stave off iron-poor blood so you'll be energized and ready to get physical in a healthy way for your mind and body. But note: If you're a vegetarian, "tea can interfere with our body's capacity to absorb non-heme iron (from plant-based foods such as beans, greens)," adds dietitian Vandana Sheth.

3 **ANXIETY (Find your balance.)** Feeling tired is a drain, but high anxiety can also be draining your energy because it's often linked to stress or depression. Welcome to feeling uneasy, muscle tension,

headaches, tired, agitated, and even to the extreme of feeling the spooky fight-or-flight response.

What Tea Rx to Use: Brew a cup by putting 1 teaspoon of black or white tea leaves into a pot of hot water. Steep for 3 minutes. For an extra calming effect, add a chamomile tea bag. Drain and serve. As you sip, close your eyes to decompress and envision yourself on a mini-trip.

Why You'll Feel Tea-rrific: The aroma and steam of a hot drink will help soothe your nerves, and your sympathetic nervous system will get a break because you are taking control and living for the moment. Pairing tea with a Mediterranean diet and lifestyle can help you chill, too. That means eat nutrient-dense whole foods, exercise, drink tea, and enjoy plain H_2O, including swimming, a hot tub, a bath, or long shower—and learn the art of relaxation (try brewing a cup of tea the British way by using a tea kettle and a teapot—making it a serene ritual).

4 **ARTHRITIS (Shake the stiffness.)** Folk medicine holds that both tea and tisanes may help anxiety woes and arthritis (painful inflammation and stiffness of the joints). Stiff and achy joints can worsen as we age (or even if we over-exercise). Arthritis is uncomfortable and can impair your movement, which can be more painful if you stop being mobile; it can be a Catch-22—if you don't use it, you'll lose it. So, it may be worth your time and effort to turn to drinking tea for easing the pain. The key to being more physical may be in your kitchen cupboard.

What Tea Rx to Use: Heat 1 cup of water in a tea kettle. Put 1 teaspoon green loose leaf tea or 1 green tea bag into a pot of hot water. Steep for 3–4 minutes and add 1 teaspoon honey. Drink a few times daily.

Why You'll Feel Tea-rrific: Black tea may lessen inflammation and arthritis pain because of its super-ingredient quercetin, a bioflavanoid that works to halt production of inflammatory chemicals in the body and lessen joint damage. Honey—any dark varietal that contains more antioxidants—also contains anti-inflammatory properties, so you'll be getting a double dose of help from nature's finest superfoods.

5 **ATHLETE'S FOOT (Zap the itch.)** Not as painful as aching joints, red, itchy, and inflamed feet is a pain in the bum and unsightly, too. Athlete's foot (at any age; I coped as a kid during swim club) is an irritating (pun intended) skin ailment often picked up by going barefoot on concrete around swimming pools and gym locker rooms. But don't despair.

What Tea Rx to Use: Infuse 4 black tea bags in 4 to 6 cups of hot water so you will get the benefits of the healing powers. Allow the tea to cool slightly until it reaches a comfortable soaking temperature. Pour it into a basin large enough to hold both feet and soak for 10 to 15 minutes. Rinse and pat dry. Repeat twice daily.

Why You'll Feel Tea-rrific: This infusion with the anti-inflammatory compounds in black tea in a foot tub can be very soothing and also help reduce the infection. Its antioxidants help reduce inflammation and when this happens it will lessen the redness and urge to scratch, which will help your feet heal faster. Plus, it's less expensive than over-the-counter creams that smell and aren't as comforting as a foot soak.

6 **BACK PAIN (Lose the throbbing.)** While athlete's foot is a contagion, an aching back, which so many cope with, can be caused by a variety of factors. These include being overweight, incurring a strain, having posture issues, tension, and whiplash from a car accident. One afternoon I was a passenger in a car when it was hit from the back and my body thrashed forward and backward. The next day, it was to the chiropractor. The diagnosis: minor whiplash, major stiffness. Doctor's orders included to keep moving, so I continued to swim. Also, to soothe my muscle tension, I drank tea.

What Tea Rx to Use: Opt for a white and black tea blend. Use 1 tea bag of each or 1 teaspoon of loose leaf of each tea in 2 cups of hot water. Steep for 3 minutes.

Why You'll Feel Tea-rrific: Both black and white tea have anti-inflammatory benefits. Also, tea proponents believe black tea increases blood flow to the brain and boosts energy. Plus, the caffeine in the tea mixture can enhance alertness. So by using the blend you'll get a nice dose of caffeine, which will give you a nudge to keep those muscles moving and therefore reduce tension. A bonus: Drinking a chamomile blend at night can help relax tight muscles.

7 **BRAIN FOG (Clear your mind!)** Burns are come and go but brain fog lingers and affects everyone sooner or later. It can be due to "burning the candle at both ends," jet lag, certain medications, or distraction by too many things going on in your life. It's a sign to get mindful like the monks in Asia centuries ago who drank tea to enjoy being Zen-like and in the now.

What Tea Rx to Use: Put one tea bag of white or black tea or 1 teaspoon of tea leaves in your teapot. Add citrus or ginseng leaves for a tastier and more mentally stimulating tea. Add 1 cup of hot water and steep for 3 minutes. Drink once or twice per day as needed.

Why You'll Feel Tea-rrific: The caffeine in white or black tea definitely can help you get and stay mindful and appreciate being in the moment. Also, ginseng is capable of "quieting the spirit, stopping agitation and enlightening the mind," as noted in a medical book during the Han dynasty. Once the mind fog lifts, it's a calming feeling to be focused on one thing, similar to decluttering your home and then sitting down and relaxing with a clear mind in a serene place.

8 **BURNS (Soothe the pain.)** Just as a sore back can be painful, so can a burn, whether it happens from touching a stovetop or a barbecue grill. The redness and inflammation of burns are painful and they can take time to heal, not to ignore the itching that follows. What to do once you feel the heat and are burned?

What Tea Rx to Use: Try a cloth soaked in white tea and place it on the red region of your skin. Repeat several times per day.

Why You'll Feel Tea-rrific: White tea is used in a variety of beauty and bath products for the skin. It contains anti-inflammatory properties that can help to soothe the redness and pain, and speed the healing process.

9 **COLDS (Warm up, baby.)** Brain fog happens year-round, but during the fall and winter months, cold season hits more frequently. Also, though, if you are under stress a cold can pay you a visit year-round, especially if traveling or contracting a virus from

someone else. If your immune system is under attack—a cold can be prevented or the severity lessened with tea.

What Tea Rx to Use: Drink one 8-ounce cup of black tea (hot or iced) with or without 1 teaspoon honey two to three times per day.

Why You'll Feel Tea-rrific: Tea researchers believe it's the compound alkylamine antigen in black tea that bolsters the body's immune system and may help guard against colds. Also, the tannins may help to stave off viruses like a cold. I recall one doctor's story about how he turned to tea for comfort. He was traveling in the Alaskan wilderness. While in a van traveling with people, one had a cold as he did. The doctor had tea and drank the liquid. And it helped the good doctor heal.

10 **CONJUNCTIVITIS (Blink away pinkeye.)** Ever have one or two red and inflamed eyes, which can affect anyone at any age? If it happens during a weekend or holiday and you can't get to the doctor, there is a way to relieve the hurt.

What Tea Rx to Use: Heat 1 cup of water and brew a black or white tea bag for 3 minutes. Drain water from bag. Place the tea bag on top of your shut eye(s) for a few minutes.

Why You'll Feel Tea-rrific: Black and white tea contain anti-inflammatory and antibacterial compounds. Not only will the tea treatment give you immediate relief, it may help prevent an infection.

11 **COUGHS (Cease the tickle.)** Coping with pinkeye can be annoying, but coughing, which can be caused by seasonal allergies, or linger after a cold, a bout of bronchitis, or other things, can be pesky and make your throat and even chest ache. In hindsight, I've experienced all three causes but springtime, when allergens including pollen, pet dander, and dust abound, is when I'm most likely to feel the urge to cough.

What Tea Rx to Use: Opt to brew 1 12-ounce cup of black or white tea. For an extra throat soother, add 1 teaspoon of honey. Repeat as needed.

Why You'll Feel Tea-rrific: Tackling a cough often takes a bit of sleuth work to discover why you are coughing—and then it's time to be proactive and deal with the problem. If allergens are the issue, for instance, it's time to get an air purifier, vacuum and dust more, and add tea with honey to your diet repertoire—soon you'll be doing the happy dance without stopping to cough.

12 **DENTAL CAVITIES (Save your teeth.)** A tickle in your throat, hacking day and night can be due to many causes and can be bothersome until nipped in the bud, but so can getting problems with your teeth. It's important to keep your mouth clean and have dental checkups twice a year with cleanings for healthy teeth and gums. You can help keep on top of the dental game by turning to tea.

What Tea Rx to Use: Try brewing 1 cup of black, white, or green tea. Do not sweeten with sugar. Drink 2 times per day, preferably in the morning and afternoon.

Why You'll Feel Tea-rrific: When you get a dental checkup twice each year, that clean bill of dental health from your hygienist and dentist will make you smile. Drinking black tea can inhibit bacteria (the stuff that increase plaque buildup). Researchers believe it's the polyphenols in this type of tea that zaps bacteria and can help keep your pearly whites cleaner and with less sticky stuff that turns into tartar and even dental decay. (If you're hesitant to drink up because of tea stains on your teeth, there are options to deter it, see chapter 18.)

13 **DEPRESSION (Lift your spirit.)** A healthy smile is healthy, but feeling down in the dumps can be nothing to smile about; it happens to most of us at one time or another during our lives. Telltale symptoms can include loss of energy and interest in doing things you like to do, sleeping too much or not enough, feeling anxious, sad, or intrusive negative thoughts. You can't just boost your mood in an instant, but—you can lift your spirit in many healthful ways including brewing a cup of tea.

What Tea Rx to Use: Opt to use the ritual of brewing tea. Pour water into the tea kettle. Once the whistle blows bring the teapot to it (rinse with hot tap water) and pour water in kettle over 2 heaping teaspoons of black tea (flavored). Steep for 3 minutes. Strain leaves. Add 1 teaspoon of honey. At night before you go to sleep, drink 1 cup of chamomile or a chamomile blend (with catnip or linden).

Why You'll Feel Tea-rrific: There are different ingredients in black tea that can boost your mood. Caffeine is a known mood-enhancer. Not only does it enhance your brainpower and get-up-and-go (getting physical can produce endorphins—the feel-good hormones like you get when you exercise, have sex, or even eat a piece of dark chocolate), but L-theanine also can help alleviate anxiety, which overlaps with depression. Caveat: After a cup or two of tea, get moving. Yes, swimming indoors/outdoors or walking outside or on the treadmill inside can help you beat anxiety and the blues by boosting the feel-good endorphins. And exercise will help balance your mood and allow you to sleep better tonight, which will help you feel better tomorrow.

14 **DERMATITIS (Heal the spots.)** Feeling low can affect your spirit, but dermatitis's red patches can irritate your skin and a rash can show on your body. As a twenty-something traveler, while visiting my grandmother in Arizona, a place of a hot, dry climate, my arms and legs had red spots on them. I didn't know what I'd caught. One doctor visit later, I was diagnosed with dermatitis. The cause could have been from sensitivity to the sun and change from a Mediterranean-type climate in the San Francisco Bay Area to a dry, Arizona desert climate.

What Tea Rx to Use: Brew a cup or two of oolong tea and drink morning and night for 1 to 2 weeks.

Why You'll Feel Tea-rrific: Research shows drinking oolong tea each day improved symptoms within a few weeks. At the end of one month, more than half of those in the study found relief. It may be that this Chinese tea contains compounds that block allergic reactions, according to scientists.[1]

15 **DIARRHEA (Stop the urge to go.)** Skin rashes aren't fun, but as our grandmothers say, "This too shall pass"—just like coping with a bout of diarrhea, often linked to bacteria caused by spoiled food, water, or even by taking a course of prescription antibiotics for a flu bug. Having a tummy ache, and having to go to the bathroom frequently, is not a vacation, especially if you're traveling.

What Tea Rx to Use: Opt to drink black or white tea combined with cinnamon. Use ½ teaspoon each of tea leaves mixed with ½ teaspoon of the herbal tea, or a tea bag of one tea and herbal tea. Heat 1 cup of water. Add 1 cinnamon tea bag. Steep for 3 minutes and add honey to taste.

Why You'll Feel Tea-rrific: Both black and white tea contain antibacterial compounds that can help destroy the germs and ease diarrhea. When I boarded a two-hour ferry ride at Long Island, California, en route to Catalina Island, I was forewarned about potential choppy water and breakers. So, I took an anti-seasickness pill. Ironically, there was no motion except in my body. By the time I arrived at the hotel room overlooking Avalon Bay, I was busy in the bathroom with a terrible case of diarrhea. Not hungry, I did drink black tea for the rest of the afternoon. The next morning I was back and enjoying frolicking in the sun, boating, swimming, and sightseeing. On the way back, I did not take any motion meds, but did drink tea before and on the boat. (I also drink tea before boarding an aircraft to counteract stomach upset if there is rough air.)

16 **DIGESTIVE WOES (Soothe your stomach.)** Bathroom problems come and go, but tummy troubles can linger. Often diet and/or stress can cause bloating, flatulence, and cramping that can take you to a specialist, as I did in college; I learned I had IBS (irritable bowel syndrome). If I could be a time traveler, I'd go back to school but change my dietary habits, not drink soda and chew gum—and turn to tea as a helper to give me relief.

What Tea Rx to Use: Try drinking 1 8-ounce cup of black tea—even better if it's infused with ginger or peppermint, two herbs that also help the stomach. Repeat two or three times daily.

Why You'll Feel Tea-rrific: Consuming black tea isn't just for diarrhea but it can be beneficial to the entire digestive tract. That means you'll be able to say good-bye to the annoyance of an inflated tummy, heartburn, and gas. Why? Give credit to the tannins in tea, which may be your heroes that help soothe intestinal distress.

17 **DIZZINESS (Feel more grounded.)** If you have experienced digestive woes, it's probably less unsettling than feeling like you're on a Tilt-a-Whirl ride and can't get off. Dizziness can

happen for many reasons including a bout of low blood sugar, side effects of medications, and even dehydration.

What Tea Rx to Use: Opt to drink 6 to 8 8-ounce glasses of water each day. This can include 2 cups of tisanes, which may be better because they do not contain caffeine.

Why You'll Feel Tea-rrific: Research shows that when our body is hydrated it performs at its optimum. If we do not get enough water—as advised in the Oldways Mediterranean Diet Pyramid—it can cause a host of physical and mental problems, not excluding feeling dizzy, which can be unsettling at best and at worst send you to the ER. So drink your water and tea to keep steady. What's more, health authorities point to tea as a noteworthy source of hydration, following water.

18 **DOWN'S SYNDROME (Getting more alert.)** Feeling unbalanced is usually a short-term unsettling symptom that can affect anyone, but Down's syndrome or Down syndrome is a long-term genetic disorder caused by an extra chromosome triggering intellectual impairment and physical abnormalities. According to research, tea may be helpful.

What Tea Rx to Use: Heat 1 cup of hot water and add 1 green tea bag or 1 teaspoon of green tea leaves. Steep for a few minutes.

Why You'll Feel Tea-rrific: A polyphenol in green tea may improve brain function by enhancing memory and behavior in people with Down syndrome, according to a study published in *The Lancet Neurology*. A year-long Spanish study, in which 43 young adults with Down syndrome were given a decaffeinated green tea supplement containing 45 percent EGCG for one year,[2] found that epigallocatechin gallate (EGCG) improved scores on memory and behavior tests. EGCG is the compound in green tea that helps lower the risk of cancer and heart disease.

19 **ENERGY DRAIN (Find your mojo.)** Mental impairment can be an obstacle, while lack of wanting to go do it, especially if you are under pressure, can be frustrating when your mind says you should do something but your body rebels and shuts down. If you are a naturally energetic person—a driven Type A personal-

ity or even Type B who likes to go have fun, without energy this can be an obstacle.

What Tea Rx to Use: Consider savoring a cup of black tea (hot or iced). Add a slice of lemon and a teaspoon of honey for an extra energy boost and flavor.

Why You'll Feel Tea-rrific: Tea proponents know black tea can get your blood circulation flowing to the brain—and that in itself can be energizing and healthier than drinking a sugary soda or energy drink with an overload of caffeine. Also, black tea is rich in good-for-you antioxidants, whereas sodas are full of empty calories.

20 EYE SKIN HYPERPIGMENTATION (Lighten up your skin.) Fighting fatigue takes some smarts, and discoloration around your eyes and eyelids is another ailment that requires trouble-shooting. I noticed the skin around my brown eyes was a light brown hue (like the copper color around my Australian shepherd's eyes). This problem can be caused by allergies and rubbing your eyes, genes, aging, and even crying.

At my dermatologist's office, the physician's assistant asked me if I had been in tears when she examined the puffy, darkened skin. My 12-year-old Brittany, Simon, recently passed and weeping was part of my grieving while coping with the loss of a soulmate with paws. The physician's assistant snapped a picture of my eyes, and left the room to show the doctor for his opinion. The background office music changed to the Simon & Garfunkel song "The Sounds of Silence." My eyes watered because of the uncanny timing—my canine companion, Simon, was monikered after one of the singers of the ageless tune—and the coincidental connection was comforting like a cup of tea.

What Tea Rx to Use: Heat water in a tea kettle, pour into a cup, and steep two white tea bags for a couple of minutes. Take out and squeeze the water from the bags. Put the bag duo in the freezer until chilled. Then, apply cold tea bags on top of your closed eyes for five or ten minutes.

Why You'll Feel Tea-rrific: The puffiness will be less noticeable. Repeat as needed. A Bonus: Add lemon juice from fresh lemon. The tannins in black tea may "tighten your skin" and "caffeine...will constrict the blood vessels," note *The Folk Remedy Encyclopedia* authors. I was told by the medical team that constant crying can interfere with the blood vessels and capillaries on the tender eye tissue. Also, I did use the juice from fresh lemons to lighten the skin. Within a few weeks, my eye tissue was almost back to normal. I blame any leftover discoloration on seasonal allergies and pool chemicals when I swim.[3]

21 **FIBROMYALGIA (Shake the aches and pains.)** Fibromyalgia is an ailment that used to be considered nonexistent or imagined by sufferers. But that has changed, and in the 21st century, medical doctors associate fibromyalgia with muscle pain, which can be paired with less energy. If you have moderate aches and pains, often stress can cause a flare-up; turning to a natural remedy may be your best bet as a first course of action.

What Tea Rx to Use: Put 1 teaspoon white tea with 1 teaspoon chamomile tea (leaves) or 1 tea bag of each in a teapot. Pour 2 cups of hot water over the tea and herbs and steep for 3 minutes. Strain, sweeten with honey, and add a bit of fresh lemon juice. Drink 1½ cups. Repeat as needed.

Why You'll Feel Tea-rrific: A small dose of caffeine (as you know, white tea has less of a kick than black tea) will give you a boost of physical and mental energy. Also, chamomile will help relax and soothe your muscles. The synergistic properties will help give you the desire to get up and move your body and refocus on action, which will help lessen your stress and boost pain-relieving endorphins (those feel-good hormones that you get when having sex or eating dark chocolate), resulting in less muscle pain. You'll feel much better, thanks to nature's tea.

22 **FLU (Say good-bye to germs.)** Dealing with aches and pains due to sensitive nerves wreaks havoc on your mind and body, as does catching the flu, which can come on suddenly, dragging you down and into bed. Viruses come in all forms and can give you anything from a 24-hour flu bug to a super bug that'll spook you to the point where images from sci-fi films like *Outbreak* and *Contagion* will haunt you as you try to shake it.

What Tea Rx to Use: Take 2 cups of tea per day and you won't be calling the doctor in the morning. Mix it up and sip 1 cup of tea (black or white) and 1 cup of your favorite vitamin C–enhanced herbal tea such as hibiscus or rooibos.

Why You'll Feel Tea-rrific: It's no surprise that the functional food tea is chock-full of antioxidants—the good guys that can keep your immune system healthy and stave off germs you could encounter anywhere from your local grocery store to a vacation stop. By drinking black tea (hot or iced) and a vitamin-rich tisane teamed with a nutrient-dense diet, you'll be keeping your immune system strong. Don't forget to exercise, de-stress, and stay clear of people who do have the flu bug to ensure you keep germ-free.

23 **FOOD POISONING (Be germ savvy.)** A bout of the stomach flu is grueling, as is eating something that can make your tummy turn topsy-turvy. Ate something that is giving your stomach trouble? My sibling got sick in Mexico despite how careful he was not to eat specific trouble-causing foods. At a movie theater I once ordered a cup of coffee. After twenty minutes into the film, my stomach began gurgling. I excused myself to the bathroom and could not leave until the title credits showed on the big screen. The coffee vendor fessed up: "I guess I didn't rinse the soap residue from the coffeepot." My stomach was gurgling, and the bathroom was my home for hours that night.

What Tea Rx to Use: Steep 2 bags of green tea or black tea in 1 cup of hot water for 3 minutes. Drink up to 2 or 3 cups daily.

Why You'll Feel Tea-rrific: Tea proponents recommend drinking strong, tannin-rich black tea to help neutralize toxins making you feel sick. Medical research in Japan revealed the catechins in green tea have an antibacterial effect, and the antioxidant may zap some E. coli and other trouble-causing bacteria.

24 **GINGIVITIS (Enjoy healthy gums.)** Not everyone experiences food poisoning, but it's not uncommon to endure inflamed gums called gingivitis at one time or another. If you want to stave off periodontal disease, take care of your gums surrounding your teeth.

What Tea Rx to Use: Drink 1 cup of black, green, or white tea combined with chamomile (½ teaspoon each of leaves or 2 bags), or green tea 2 to 3 times per day until inflammation is gone. Also, you can put a wet tea bag on your gums (often there are trouble spots around crowns or an area you haven't flossed well).

Why You'll Feel Tea-rrific: This cost-effective tea and tisane home cure can calm inflamed gum tissue thanks to the anti-inflammatory and antibacterial properties in tea and herbal teas like chamomile. That means the ache and puffy gums may subside. Not only will you be out of pain, but maintaining healthy gums is part of preserving your pearly whites for a lifetime. Here's proof: In a study showing promising results, nearly 1,000 Japanese men, aged 49 to 59 years old, took part in a health exam. Those who drank one cup of green tea per day had gums that were healthier than those who drank less green tea.[4]

What's more, it's no surprise that tea's positive effect on oral health is due to antioxidants—mighty catechins and their healing powers. Researchers advise drinking 2 to 3 cups on a daily basis.[5]

25 **HOT FLASHES (Cool down fast.)** Tea can help keep your gums healthy, especially during high stress times in life—and that includes going through a few hot flashes during and after menopause! During my PMS-ing days as a health journalist I'd write articles about the pause but couldn't relate to a "hot flash."

What Tea Rx to Use: Drink iced tea daily. Green tea or white tea works well, either a tea bag or leaves is advised. Repeat as needed.

Why You'll Feel Tea-rrific: While hot flashes (not common in China or Japan, where women drink green tea) are not something that will be the end of you, they can be unsettling. One time at a book signing a flash out of nowhere came to my table. My face turned bright red and I was happy for the layered look as I removed a neck scarf, sweater, and top. But probably the best remedy was the cup of hot green tea that was brought to my table—it had an instant calming and cooling effect.

26 **INSECT BITES (Treat the hurt.)** Irregularity is not a big problem for me, because I follow the "rules" above but my life in the mountains brings a new challenge. I've had my share of insect

bite escapades, including an *Arachnophobia* film–like incident with a wolf spider from the firewood pile I brought into the cabin. The spider bite on my cheek required a doctor's visit and tetanus shot; both arm and cheek ached and were swollen for two days. But tea compresses may have helped the hurt.

What Tea Rx to Use: Try heating a cup of water and soaking a black or white tea bag for a few minutes. Put the moist tea bag on top of the area. Repeat 3–4 times daily.

Why You'll Feel Tea-rrific: Tea contains anti-inflammatory and antibacterial properties—both can help calm the redness and swollen skin. Also, drinking a few cups of antioxidant-rich tea during this time will bolster your immune system to help fight off a potential infection, and drinking tea can help calm frazzled nerves from Mother Nature's scourge of insect bites.

27 **INSOMNIA (Get your shut-eye.)** An insect's bite can interrupt your daily bliss, but so can insomnia—the inability to fall asleep (think of the memorable film *Insomnia*, when actor Al Pacino cannot sleep due to the never-ending northern light of Alaska in the summertime). Not getting adequate shut-eye can affect your mood and body because we need sleep to help rejuvenate and renew our immune system. Decaffeinated tea can come to the rescue but so can some herbal teas.

What Tea Rx to Use: Put herbal tea leaves of ½ teaspoon catnip, ½ teaspoon linden, ½ teaspoon chamomile into 2 cups hot water. Steep for 3–5 minutes, strain. Drink 12 ounces a few hours before bedtime.

Why You'll Feel Tea-rrific: Catnip, linden, and chamomile are well-known sleep enhancers due to the calming properties in the "nervine" type herbs. Tea master Daniel Johnson agrees and knows chamomile and mint work together and "calm the mind." He says, "Mindfully enjoying it at nighttime can provide us an opportunity to reflect upon our day and let go of any stressful experiences. It is my favorite tea to drink in the evening as an herbal 'nightcap.'" The sleep-inducing beverage is "complemented by a sweet drizzle of local honey," adds Johnson.

28 **INTERSTITIAL CYSTITIS (Ease the discomfort.)** While not being able to get shut-eye, inflammation of the bladder is not

uncommon but it is often a pain for both women and men. Stress, trigger foods, and not staying hydrated all can cause a flare-up. The symptoms can include going to the bathroom too much (or feeling an urge to do so), pelvic pain, and discomfort.

What Tea Rx to Use: Try drinking 1 cup of chamomile herbal tea. Follow with an 8-ounce glass of water. Repeat as necessary.

Why You'll Feel Tea-rrific: Chamomile is recommended because it can calm your nerves and it is a natural anti-inflammatory. During a bout of cystitis, you want to stay clear of caffeinated teas. Sometimes they can be a trigger for IC sufferers—but not always—as long as consumed in moderation and along with regular water intake. The more relaxed you are, the more you'll feel at ease and your cystitis will go away.

29 **IRREGULARITY (Finding your routine.)** Dealing with hot flashes is flustering, but when chronic constipation pays you untimely visits, it comes with plenty of symptoms including bloat, discomfort, and sluggishness. Welcome to constipation, which can be caused by not drinking enough water, lack of exercise, not eating enough fiber, some prescription medications, and even traveling, which upsets your daily routine.

What Tea Rx to Use: Heat 1 cup of water and add 2 black tea bags. Steep for 3 minutes. Repeat 2 to 3 times per day.

Why You'll Feel Tea-rrific: Caffeine can help stimulate your body's system and help you get back on the regular track just as a cup of joe can do. Since black tea contains more caffeine than green and white tea, it's the choice of tea for irregularity. Herbal teas added to black tea may even give you an added boost. When I had been traveling for one week in British Columbia, Canada, due to the late-night flight and early-morning train, and sporadic eating, my regular bathroom schedule was off. Back in Seattle I was on a trek through Pike Place; my mission was to find prunes. Mission unaccomplished, I left, and made a cup of strong black tea. Twenty minutes later, tea came to the rescue. I was regular once again and energetic for the trip back home.

30 **IRRITABILITY: (Calm your nerves.)** Chronic cystitis is a bear to face, but feeling touchy or ill-tempered isn't fun for you or people in your life. A variety of things can cause you to be grouchy,

including out-of-whack hormones, relationship and financial worries, or perhaps seasonal change. Of course, no functional food can fix obstacles for you but tea can help you to cope a bit better as you go along the journey of life.

What Tea Rx to Use: Use ½ teaspoon each of chamomile and lavender leaves in 1 cup of boiling water. Drink as needed.

Why You'll Feel Tea-rrific: As a loyal fan of chamomile tea (both tea bags and loose leaf), I am a convert to chamomile blends. This concoction is one I tried from Cal-a-Vie Spa Specialty Tea—and I was amazed at how calm I felt after savoring a cup of the brew. Tea proponents will tell you herbal teas, like these herbs, may help sleepless nights, mood swings from hormonal woes, or if you just have had one of those challenging days. A flavonoid in chamomile, apigenin, is believed to influence receptors in the brain that help relax nerves and tight muscles. Other herbs used in herbal teas contain antioxidants, too, and do their magic. (See chapter 11, "Healing Herbal Teas.")

31 JET LAG (Snag some energy.) When you travel it's not uncommon for your erratic schedule to interfere with your body's biological clock, or circadian rhythm. Catching an early morning flight at 6:00 A.M. (at the airport two hours before) and flying a long flight, or catching an early morning train or ferry to your destination can all end up in a case of jet lag.

What Tea Rx to Use: Drink 1 cup of white tea before an early morning flight. Chase it later in the day with 1 cup of black or green tea. Repeat as necessary.

Why You'll Feel Tea-rrific: Drinking white tea in the early morning hours is better on your system than a cup of joe or black tea because the former has less caffeine but enough to wake you up so you'll be alert. Savoring a stronger cup of tea later in the day can help you feel awake and energized but not as much as coffee, which can leave you feeling jittery.

32 KIDNEY STONES (Hydrate, hydrate, hydrate.) The pain of kidney stones is something you don't want to come visit you. I recall a male friend who dealt with this health issue and the treatments weren't anything you'd cherish.

What Tea Rx to Use: Opt for at least two cups of tea—any type will suffice—per day.

Why You'll Feel Tea-rrific: Past research shows that upping your water intake, including tea, can help lessen the risk of kidney stones. Evidently not consuming adequate water can be one reason why these babies develop—whether you are male or female. A study that followed more than 80,000 women for nearly one decade showed that for each 8-ounce cup of tea consumed each day by the women—who had no history of kidney stones—the risk of developing stones may be lowered by 8 percent.[6]

Tea Romance for One: Afternoon Delight

Tea is romantic and tea in the afternoon is as good as it gets. Let me share a memory of tea and chocolate in Seattle. . . .

Upon returning from British Columbia I stopped in Seattle for the afternoon and nighttime. My favorite hotel room at the Grand Hyatt Seattle was reserved for me. On the 29th floor, I was in tea heaven stowed away in the Emerald Suite with a panoramic view of Puget Sound, enjoying 800 square feet of panoramic bliss and tea(s).

At first, it was my desire to leave my bags in this breathtaking room and take a walk downtown. I stopped at Pike Place Market overlooking the Elliott Bay waterfront and strolled through the stores. It was raining when I walked toward the ferries—"One day I will go to Victoria," I mumbled. I walked up and down the sidewalks and stopped at Starbucks. "A small mocha and petite vanilla scone," I ordered. When I sat down with my treats I felt a sense of homesickness and the Sierra in the fall.

At a hair styling shop where I was a looking for a conditioner for my locks that frizz in rainy weather, the stylist said: "If I were staying at your hotel, I'd be there—not walking around in this weather." I responded: "Gosh, you're right." I grabbed my bag and hiked back to the Hyatt. Up the elevator I went to the high floor—the room with a view, per my request, the third time I've stayed; the doorman remembered me. When I put my bag on the desk in the study my heart stopped. I exhaled. The concierge remembered my birthday. In front of me was a white ceramic teapot, cup, and an array of tea bags. Next to the tea display gourmet chocolate truffles and bars greeted me. I was grateful and excited. I poured myself a cup of tea, plopped on the bed, and admired my spacious room, as well as the panoramic view of the great Pacific Northwest. I turned on a film and ordered dinner—a grilled cheese and fries. As I waited for my comfort food, I took in the luxury of it all. I thought: "I'm in heaven. This room is my home away from home." If there is a tea heaven—I had arrived. It was a romantic birthday for one.

33 **MEMORY LAPSES (Find that thought.)** Libido can wax and wane depending on your mood, environment, relationship, and work. Forgetting things such as where you put your keys or an appointment can be due to causes like doing too much or having a senior moment. Everyone one time or another will allow something to slip their mind but it doesn't mean you are losing it—just a temporary moment.

What Tea Rx to Use: Drink 1 cup of strong black tea (use leaves or a bag) or ginseng. Forget sugar. Repeat as needed.

Why You'll feel Tea-rrific: Tea studies show that certain compounds are doing their job when it comes to enhancing short-term memory. This is due in part to tea's pro-mental function properties such as L-theanine—a compound that can boost alpha waves and cognitive function.

34 **MORNING SICKNESS (Baby your tummy.)** A decrease in libido due to feeling kind of seasick in the A.M. hours is the scourge of pregnancy countless women can and do experience. Feeling queasy to nauseated is anything but sexy and can be very uncomfortable. In the 20th century, pregnant women often nibbled on saltine crackers; but during this century many have found that morning sickness may be prevented or made less severe if a mother-to-be turns to tea—as fishermen did and do.

What Tea Rx to Use: Opt to heat 1 cup of water. Add 1 heaping teaspoon of ginger leaves or a ginger tea bag. Steep. Drain. Add a bit of honey to taste.

Why You'll Feel Tea-rrific: Gingerroot is touted by herbalists to help ease tummy trouble. Research shows that it can help. Past studies decades ago have shown ginger (capsules, cookies, and tea) can help lessen the side effects of motion sickness.

35 **MUSCLE SPASMS (Stop the twitching.)** Ah, a troubled tummy is one plight, but a muscle spasm that happens out of nowhere is also a challenge. Imagine your leg or side tightening and you do not have control of the uneasy feeling.

What Tea Rx to Use: Prepare a blend of premium chamomile herbal tea and white tea. Use ½ teaspoon each of leaves. Heat water in a tea kettle, pour into a ceramic pot. Steep for 3 minutes. Repeat as necessary.

Why You'll Feel Tea-rrific: It is believed that drinking chamomile tea raises urine levels of glycine, a compound that calms muscle spasms. So this is one perk of why this herbal tea could prove to be an effective home remedy for pesky menstrual cramps.

36 **PLANTAR WARTS (Lose the lump.)** Small bumps on the fingers or on the bottom of your foot can be unsightly and hurt, too. While these warts are commonplace at any age, they can be stubborn. Worse, even if you pay the dermatologist to remove the warts—it is painful with dry ice or other methods—they may return. So what to do?

What Tea Rx to Use: Heat one cup of water and add 2 black tea bags. Steep for several minutes. Apply tea with cotton ball on wart. Repeat several times per day. You can include a bit of manuka honey vinegar to expedite healing.

Why You'll Feel Tea-rrific: The tannins in the black tea paired with acetic acid in honey will help dry up the wart thanks to the anti-inflammatory properties. It hurts less than having an invasive procedure done at a doctor's office or some of the over-the-counter type of liquids that can burn and ache during and after applying it.

37 **PMS (Pamper those symptoms.)** Warts are temporary, as is premenstrual syndrome. Women in their teens until their early fifties face and survive monthly symptoms of premenstrual syndrome with a mixed bag of spooky symptoms. The most common woes include cramps, crankies, and cravings, which can lead to overindulging in sweets and end up in weight gain. Tea can come to the rescue.

What Tea Rx to Use: Heat 2 cups of water. Brew 1 teaspoon each of white tea (its lower caffeine content will take the edge off rather than using black or green tea) and calming chamomile. Add a slice of citrus and a bit of honey to taste.

Why You'll Feel Tea-rrific: Not only will the hot cup of tea soothe your irritability, the white tea and chamomile tea will help lessen cramps and calm your muscles. A bonus effect: The honey curbs the urge to eat sweets and can help boost your energy and mood.

38 **POISON OAK/IVY (Lose the itch.)** Premenstrual syndrome is not life-threatening but the unpredictable symptoms can feel like it's a party spoiler, not unlike poison oak. As a tween, I got poison oak from hiking in the hills when it rained and showering afterward. By the morning I had a terrible case of poison oak—blisters and red patches on my hands, arms, and face. In the 20th century, the remedy was calamine lotion but today, I would turn to tea.

What Tea to Use: Apply a wet black or white tea bag on the red patches of your skin. Repeat several times per day.

Why You'll Feel Tea-rrific: The tea bag with its antioxidant compounds will help relieve itching and redness and speed up the healing process. Not only will it bring instant results, the treatment is clear and not messy like messy lotions.

39 **SEASONAL AFFECTIVE DISORDER (Blast the blues.)** Patience for poison oak to run its course is challenging, but feeling down and sluggish with seasonal affective disorder (SAD), coined by Dr. Norman Rosenthal, is another monster to face. After writing numerous articles on this topic, I have tackled the symptoms with an arsenal of remedies—and tea is on the list come late fall through early spring.

What Tea Rx to Use: Brew 1 cup of hot water and use 1 teaspoon green tea leaves or tea bag. Steep for 3 minutes. Repeat 2 times per day.

Why You'll Feel Tea-rrific: One man in his forties told me in the afternoon before going back to work, especially during the colder winter months, he'd feel tired, agitated, and just wanted to go home and crawl into bed. But he vowed that ordering a 16-ounce cup of China Green Tips at a local coffee shop changed his mood. "I can't believe this tea is legal!" he exclaimed. I looked up the nutritional benefits and the large tea has 45 milligrams of caffeine (which can give you a physical and mental burst of energy). But also, green tea contains L-theanine—a compound that enhances brain chemicals including serotonin and that can give you a calming sense of well-being like antidepressants do—and these perks can help you to eat less and lose unwanted pounds.

40 **SINUSITUS (Baby your sinuses.)** Sensing the scourge of seasonal changes isn't uncommon, nor is a bout of sinusitis. Feeling congested? Got postnasal drip? Or is that headache between your eyes bothering you? Join the club—and it's more common for sinusitis to pay you a visit during seasonal changes, including fall and spring.

What Tea Rx to Use: Opt to sip a 12-ounce cup of freshly brewed white or black tea—flavored varieties are fine, too (with a teaspoon each of apple cider vinegar and honey). Repeat as needed daily.

Why You'll Feel Tea-rrific: The hot water helps to decongest your sinuses, keep you hydrated, and lessening postnasal drip in the throat. Both vinegar and honey contain ingredients to help with inflammation of your sinuses, which can alleviate the facial pain, toothaches, and that headache, too.

41 **SORE THROAT (Treat the pain.)** Sinus symptoms come and go, and sometimes come with a scratchy, raspy throat. Also, before a cold you can get a telltale sore throat. Not to forget allergies and even talking too much. Rather than run to the doctor for an allergy medication, why not take an alternative route and turn to tea?

What Tea Rx to Use: Dried green or oolong tea leaves combined with rose hips or hibiscus can be a perfect pairing. Put 1 teaspoon of tea leaves and 1 teaspoon of the herbal tea of your choice in 1 cup of hot water. Steep for a few minutes, then strain. Add honey to taste.

Why You'll Feel Tea-rrific: Oolong tea and green tea may reduce swelling and inflammation, due its flavonoids. Also, honey boasts anti-inflammatory benefits, too. When I am a guest on national radio, I often take 1 tablespoon of honey with anti-inflammatory chamomile tea before I'm on-air. It takes away the hoarseness (usually due to allergies or talking too much) and my voice sounds soothing without that cackle.

42 **STOMACHACHE (Soothe the queasies.)** A sore throat isn't any more welcome than an upset stomach. A stomachache can be triggered by a variety of factors including eating something that doesn't agree with you, motion sickness (car, boat, or plane) or even a bout of the stomach flu. No matter the reason, you'll want a remedy to beat feeling nauseated.

What Tea Rx to Use: Tummy Soothing Chamomile-Ginger Tea: Combine 1 teaspoon ginger tea and 1 teaspoon chamomile tea (tea bag or leaves). Heat 2 cups tap water in a tea kettle. Add tea in strainer for 3–5 minutes. Add a slice of orange and honey to taste. This is an easy, all-natural rescue remedy. Makes 2 servings.

Why You'll Feel Tea-rrific: Both chamomile and ginger contain properties that can help stave off tummy distress. Calming chamomile can stave off anxiety (stomach distress is a symptom) and ginger is touted for its compounds to beat nausea. I recall one day in between book signings, I was with the late geologist Jim Berkland. We went on a drive before the Walnut Creek Barnes & Noble event. He was fearless, excited to drive up Mount Diablo, pointing out all the rock formations. But a strong stomach is required to stomach twists and turns on that winding road. That night, Jan, his wife, exclaimed: "Jim! You didn't take Callie up that road, did you?" She fed me oatmeal cookies and chamomile tea, which calmed my stomach. (See the "Herbal Teas" chapter for more about these two herbs and their healing powers.)

43 STOMACH ULCERS (Stop the burning.) A stomachache goes away but an ulcer can return. Either can be bothersome—but blame stomach ulcers on *Helicobacter pylori* or bacteria. I remember a few people in my life who said they had a gastric ulcer. One girlfriend used to drink milk and said it coated her ulcers. I'm wondering now if she had sipped a cup of tea or two daily that perhaps those ulcers would have been history.

What Tea Rx to Use: Brew 1 cup of Darjeeling (a black tea) or white tea. Drink once or twice daily, especially during times when you sense a flare-up.

What You'll Feel Tea-rrific: Antibiotics can be a course of action to deal with gastric ulcers. However, research shows tea may one day be the prescription of choice, too. A variety of tea extracts may inhibit bacteria growth in ulcers. But further studies are needed before your doctor will prescribe tea as the cure-all medicine of choice for ulcer relief.

44 STRESS (Disconnect and decompress.) Tummy trouble happens to all of us once in a while, as does stress overload. Common stressors from work and financial problems to major life changes such as divorce or loss of a loved one can take a toll on your mind, body, and spirit. Constant stress without a tea break, however, can weaken your immune system and may cause poor lifestyle choices, leaving your body more vulnerable to colds, infections, and even heart disease.

What Tea Rx to Use: One 8-ounce cup of English Breakfast tea, a black tea that may help you to chill. Add a slice of lemon and/or a bit of honey to intensify the calming antidote.

Why You'll Feel Tea-rrific: According to researchers, an amino acid called L-theanine compound found in black tea, in combination with caffeine, might lessen stress hormones such as cortisol, which can help induce a calmer feeling and increase mood. Researchers discovered how this black tea can help you to chill faster. The study was done at the University College in London and published in the *Journal of Psychopharmacology*.[7]

45 SUMMER BLUES (Snap out of it.) Depression can rise in the wintertime for people who are seasonal affective disorder suffer-

ers. But summer can also affect serotonin levels, making you feel down, especially if you live in a region when the heat soars. Or if you live in a tourist town and the quietude is suddenly changed to a hectic environment with loud noises, traffic, and crowded stores, all of which can wreak havoc on your nerves.

What Tea Rx to Use: Opt to try a blend of black and white or green and white tea. Use 1 teaspoon of each or 1 bag of each and 2 cups of water. Heat to almost a boil; steep for 3 minutes. Drain. Serve with calming citrus slices.

Why You'll Feel Tea-rrific: Both white and green tea have less caffeine than black tea—but all three teas boast calming effects. Drinking a hot cup of tea in the morning or night or iced tea throughout the day can also beat stress and calm your frazzled nerves.

46 SUNBURN (Treat your skin.) Summer can be a drag for some people, especially fair-skinned winter lovers who detest getting burned by the sun. My sibling, blue-eyed with a light Irish complexion like my father, for instance, traveled to Cabo, Mexico, a place touted for its warm climate. He went fishing and enjoyed the water and sun all day long on a chartered boat. Unwittingly, his legs and feet were not covered with a sunscreen. The damage was second-degree burns that sent him to a general practitioner once he arrived back home to California.

What Tea Rx to Use: Cool a strong infusion of white tea, use it to soak a sponge or soft cloth, and then gently pat onto sunburned skin. Infused tea can also be added to a spray bottle or atomizer to apply without touching painful burns, according to *The Everything Healthy Tea Book.* Or, if your legs and arms are suffering from a sunburn (which can hurt a lot; it happened to me in Las Vegas after sunbathing by a pool too long), try a cool bath with white tea–infused water.

Why You'll Feel Tea-rrific: Whether you are away or at home, tea is an inexpensive, soothing treatment that can offer immediate relief as well as continue to work to soothe the pain, redness, and inflammation of a sunburn, thanks to the compounds found in antioxidant-rich white tea—often used in beauty skin products.

47 **TMJ (Relax yourself, baby.)** Dental issues can include problems with your temporomandibular joint (TMJ), which connects your jawbone to your skull. Personally, I have been tested by my dentist for a TMJ disorder—it can cause aching in one or both your jaw joints and in the muscles that control your jaw movement. But I flunked . . . If you, however, pass the test and are diagnosed with TMJ, you aren't doomed to jaw pain for life. Often, symptoms of TMJ (linked to poor posture, stress, and even eating hard foods) can make the pain of sore teeth, or the jawbone, and even the inability to open your mouth a debilitating ailment to face. But you're hardly alone and there is help.

What Tea Rx to Use: Brew one cup of hot water. Add 1 teaspoon or one tea bag of herbal tea such as chamomile or lavender. Repeat two to three times daily, especially before bedtime.

Why You'll Feel Tea-rrific: One you get a handle on destressing and coping with day-to-day stressors in life, odds are higher if your TMJ is mild you may see that the symptoms will pass. Calming teas can affect your nervous system in a healing way just as prescription medications can do. If you're on an even keel and living life in a more grounded way, your days of a sore mouth may be history.

48 **TOOTH PROCEDURES (Tend to your pearly whites.)** Coping with a sunburn from being out in the sun too long is hard, but dealing with dental issues is no picnic either. Unfortunately, I've been dealt both at different times—and it seems that both challenges can be helped with tea. I recall my dentist used to offer hot water in a coffee container for patients to drink black tea in his San Francisco office waiting room. And now I know why he may have done just that.

Tea Rx to Use: Drink 1 8-ounce cup of black tea or white tea. Repeat two times per day, preferably in the morning and afternoon.

Why You'll Feel Tea-rrific: Tea researchers believe black tea not only can inhibit bacteria growth in the mouth, but sipping a cup of tea can also offer a sense of tranquility that is helpful when you're having a crown procedure to save a back molar, or having a front tooth bonded to preserve the tooth and be aesthetically pleasing.

49 **UNIVERSAL EMERGENCY (Get prepared, not scared.)** Problems with a sore jaw can feel like a major catastrophe in your life, but once you take action and contact your dentist for preventive measures to follow, you'll find it often is a temporary ailment. But being blindsided by an untimely event, such as a major earthquake, hurricane, or wildfire, is much worse. Imagine: You have minutes—or not—to grab a few of your belongings, including a first-aid kit, and get the heck out of Dodge. Or stay put. Either way, having tea(s) on hand in time of disaster can be a godsend if you need an energetic boost or brainpower or must endure a cut, stomachache, frazzled nerves, or even dry skin.

What Tea Rx to Use: Put boxes of tea such as black and white, and calming chamomile or lavender herbal teas into an airtight container; store these tea products with your emergency supplies.

Why You'll Feel Tea-rrific: If you experience an emergency, tea is a universal item that can be used both internally and externally. That means, it can help keep a cut from getting infected thanks to its anti-inflammatory properties; it can also benefit you via its ingredients to calm frazzled nerves. During a natural or man-made disaster, tea and tisanes just may be the essential lifesaver that you'll be glad you packed away for emergency preparedness. Drinking tea—black and white—can help boost the immune system, which is vital during a stressful event, and lower the risk of heart disease (yes, it calms and that can keep your blood pressure from skyrocketing). Also, herbal teas—lemon balm and linden—can help relieve insomnia. Tisanes are the ultimate cure-all in time of need and should be part of your first-aid kit in the home, office, and car.

50 **WARTS (Lose those bumps.)** Common skin warts are not an emergency, but these pesky, harmless lumps often found on the hands are not easy on the eyes. Instead of running to the dermatologist and deal with freezing to cutting, first try using a natural remedy for a less invasive touch.

What Tea Rx to Use: Mix one part strong brewed black tea (leaves are suggested to get more antioxidant power) with one part apple cider vinegar on a cotton ball or tissue and apply several times daily to the wart. Repeat until the wart is gone.

Why You'll Feel Tea-rrific: Superfood tea and vinegar proponents believe it's the tannic acid in tea and acetic acid in vinegar—those mighty antioxidants—that can help get rid of the wart. I can attest that vinegar does work (it took one week for a wart on the hand; a few weeks for a wart on the sole of my foot); I would add tea if ever challenged again by these little troublemakers on the skin before running to the doctor.

A BONUS TEA CURE: WEIGHT WOES (Stop mindless overeating.) Bulimia is a weighty dilemma that can affect both women and men. It's a problem when people have a bad body image of themselves. Thus, they will turn to bingeing on food to fill a void and it becomes a cycle. It's a mental issue, but also a body issue that can be helped with a nutrient-rich diet, exercise, and counseling—and tea during the day and night may also be helpful.

What Tea to Use: Use 1 teaspoon dried chamomile leaves (a blend with catnip and linden is good) in 1 cup of hot water. Steep for about 4 minutes. Drink 2 times daily.

Why You'll Feel Tea-rrific: Calming chamomile has properties that can soothe a busy mind and help you to stay balanced and feel more centered. Once you are in a mindful set, and a living-for-the-moment place, "what-ifs" and other intrusive, negative self-talk may be lessened and a more positive frame of mind may come into play. "It fills you up and helps with your hydration," adds dietitian Vandana Sheth. She adds, "Sometimes when you are thirsty we may mistake thirst for hunger." By sipping a comforting cuppa you may stave off the urge to reach for food that you really do not want to eat. But then, there are times when your sweet tooth pays you a visit and you can savor treats in moderation to keep you from overindulging.

Lemon Custard Tart

Lemon and tea pair like apple pie and vanilla ice cream. Years ago, my friend Gemma Sciabica created a special "Biscottea" recipe for me. It called for a store-bought lemon pudding cake mix. I made the call to switch it to her lemon tarts—a healthier treat included on tearoom menus.

Use 1 tart crust for a 10-inch fluted tart pan with a removable bottom.

FILLING

1 cup milk
¾ cup sugar
½ cup lemon or lime juice
4 eggs, large
2 tablespoons corn starch
2 tablespoons lemon or lime peel
1 tablespoon Marsala olive oil
¼ teaspoon salt

Preheat oven to 350 degrees. In mixing bowl whisk together milk, sugar, lemon juice, eggs, corn starch, lemon peel, olive oil, and salt. Pour into tart crust, bake 50 minutes or until set. Serves approximately 8.

(Author's Note: I topped each tart with a dollop of homemade whipped cream and 2 tablespoons fresh blueberries.) Serve with black or white tea.

(*Courtesy: Baking Sensational Sweets with California Olive Oil* by Gemma Sanita Sciabica.)

In chapter 16, "Beau-tea-ful Possibilities," you'll find out about the best brews—that go back centuries—to use both inside and outside your body for feeling and looking beautiful.

TEA-CENTRIC HEALING HINTS TO STEEP

If it doesn't specify which form or variety of tea to use, go ahead and use your own preference.

Ailment	Tea	What It May Do
✓ Allergies	Green, white tea and local honey	Relieve sneezing, congestion
✓ Anemia	Dandelion, raspberry herbal tea	Boost red blood cells
✓ Anxiety	Chamomile tea	Soothes frazzled nerves
✓ Arthritis	Green tea	Relaxes muscles and stiff joints
✓ Athlete's foot	Black tea	Dries and heals irritation and itchy skin
✓ Back pain	White and black tea	Relaxes muscles so you will get moving
✓ Brain fog	Black tea	Stimulates brainpower
✓ Burns	Black tea	Soothes smarting, inflammation
✓ Colds	Black tea or red berry herbal teas	May speed recovery
✓ Conjunctivitis	Black or white tea	Soothes inflammation, redness
✓ Cough	Black or white tea	Soothes tickle
✓ Dental caries	White or green tea	Staves off plaque buildup and bacteria
✓ Depression	Black tea	Boosts mood
✓ Dermatitis	Oolong tea	Heals redness, inflammation
✓ Diarrhea	Black or white tea	Helps regulate bowel movements

✓ Digestive problems	Black tea	Soothes stomach upset
✓ Dizziness	Tea or tisanes	Aids in feeling centered or grounded
✓ Down's syndrome	Green tea	Stimulates mental alertness
✓ Energy drain	Black tea	Boosts energy levels
✓ Eye skin pigmentation	White tea and lemon	Lightens brownish areas
✓ Fibromyalgia	Chamomile or white tea	Lessens aches and pains and relaxes muscles
✓ Flu	Black or white tea	Speeds recovery with rooibos, rose hips
✓ Food poisoning	Black or green tea	Eliminates bacteria
✓ Gingivitis	Black tea, chamomile tea	Soothes inflamed gums
✓ Hot flashes	Green tea	Maintains normal temperatures
✓ Insect bites	Black tea	Heals inflammation
✓ Insomnia	Chamomile, lavender tea	Aids relaxation, sleep
✓ Interstitial cystitis	Chamomile tea	Relaxes, soothes muscles
✓ Irregularity	Tea	Aids in chronic constipation
✓ Irritability	Chamomile tea	Calms nerves, agitation
✓ Jet lag	White tea	Aids biological clock
✓ Kidney stones	Tea or non-teas	Helps increase water intake
✓ Memory lapses	Black or ginseng tea	Boosts brainpower
✓ Morning sickness	Ginger tea	Helps queasiness

✓ Muscle cramps	White tea	Relaxes nervous system
✓ Plantar's wart	Black tea	Dries up wart
✓ PMS	White tea	Lessens cramps, crankies
✓ Poison oak/ivy	Black and white teas	Stops itching, aids redness
✓ Seasonal affective disorder	Black or green tea	Boosts mood, energy, lessens simple carb cravings
✓ Sinusitis	Black or white tea	Relieves stuffed-up nasal passages
✓ Sore throat	Chamomile tea and honey	Soothes soreness, irritation
✓ Stomachache	Rose hips tisane	Aids in queasiness
✓ Stomach ulcers	Darjeeling or white tea	Soothes pain, heals
✓ Stress	English Breakfast tea	Calms nervous system
✓ Summer blues	Green and white tea	Boosts energy and mood enhancer
✓ Sunburn	White tea	Soothes redness and burning
✓ Tooth procedures	Black or white tea	Destresses and calms gum tissue
✓ TMJ	Chamomile and lavendar tisanes	Calms nervous system
✓ Universal emergency	Black, white, green teas, herbal teas	Acts as cure-all
✓ Warts	Tea with vinegar	Rids of lumps and bumps
✓ Weight woes	Chamomile tea	Calms nerves, lessens mindless overeating

PART 7

FUTURE TEA

Beau-tea-ful Possibilities

Stands the Church clock at ten to three?
And is there honey still for tea?
   —Rupert Brooke, *The Old Vicarage, Grantchester*

After arriving in Montréal, after a 3,000-mile flight, I ended up at my Montréal Marriott Chateau Champlain hotel room at 2:00 A.M. I was pleasantly surprised by the half-moon window overlooking a picture-perfect view of downtown Montréal. As tired as I was, a fresh cup of chamomile tea was in my hands while admiring the city skyline before I fell asleep.

When I awoke, at 9:00 A.M., I noticed the courtesy fresh fruit basket while brewing a cup of black tea. I called room service and ordered: fresh fruit and a waffle. While I drew a bath, the array of bath and beauty products grabbed my attention. The bar soaps were infused with lavender and rosemary—two herbs I've used in tea cuisine. It was early fall, and a chilly 10 degrees outside. A hot bath, fresh tea, and herbal beauty amenities made me feel at home despite the fact that I was not on the West Coast, but in Canada, a place I ran away from when I was in my twenties because of the novelty. Now, like a pampered princess with natural beauty items, a bath, stimulating tea—and a new city to explore—I was in heaven and out of my comfort zone in a French-speaking province.

THE BEAU-TEA OF TEA POWER

If you think luxury hotels, like this one, and posh health spas do not serve tea, think again. Today's spas, complete with spa-infused treatment menus, are pricey but some regimens are cut in time and can be budget-friendly. And more people—both women and men—are discovering the beauty of being pampered with tea.

It's no beauty secret that drinking tea can enhance your blood circulation, zaps stress and anxiety, and hydrates your skin from head to toe. Cal-a-Vie, north of San Diego, California, offers the same teas I include in *The Healing Powers of Tea*. Black teas, white teas, green teas, red teas, and herbal teas are found at this destination spa, thanks to the Spa Signature Teas by Special Tea Company. The array of tea blends perfectly reflects the combination of California ideas of fitness, European spa philosophies, and healthy nutrition for the body and spirit that spas like this one provide.

Getting spa'd by savoring teas *or* enjoying tea-infused beauty treatments from head to toe (literally) that are offered at other luxury health spas including Canyon Ranch, which is located in Tucson, Arizona, and in the Berkshire Mountains of Massachusetts, has been popular for decades and is likely to be an ongoing trend.

The thing is, if you are traveling or lucky to live in a region nearby a spa with tea-infused beauty treatments, you've hit the jackpot. If not, let me show you some of the delights on a typical spa treatment menu—you can go do it—or duplicate it yourself. (I will show you how to do just that.)

TEA-INFUSED SPA BEAUTY TREATMENTS MENU

Here, take a look at some of the popular head-to-toe beauty treatments on spa menus around the globe at five-star hotels. Since spa regimens change, here is a sample, much like a box of fine chocolates—you may be pleasantly surprised.

Green Tea Age-Defying Facial—promises to help lessen signs of aging and help repair sun damage.

Green Tea Face and Body Refresher—green tea and notes of citrus with a facial, followed by aromatherapy massage for hands, arms, legs, and feet.

Green Tea and Ginger Mud Body Mask—starts with a grapeseed body scrub followed by a mud made with green tea that is smoothed on the body to cleanse, detoxify the skin. A gingerroot moisturizer is then applied to invigorate skin and help muscle aches and pains.

White Tea and Avocado Body Scrub—a full-body massage with the anti-aging white tea and good-for-you oils in avocado to hydrate paired with a cup of white tea.

LUXURY HOTELS OFFER TEA-INFUSED BEAUTY AND BATH COLLECTIONS

While I traveled from Montréal, Quebec, to Vancouver, the herbal bath items were a prelude to more beauty and bath product lines I would later discover when I traveled again to both British Columbia, Canada, and Seattle, Washington. I noticed other luxury hotels provide tea-infused products to their patrons.

Hyatt Hotels: Hyatt Hotel guests can receive the beauty and bath benefits of June Jacobs Spa Collection—Green Tea & Cucumber products, including body balm, cleansing bar, purifying shower gel, and toner. The blend of antioxidant-rich white, red, and green tea extracts may help soothe your skin and make your stay at the Hyatt feel like a day at the spa. (I have the Green Tea & Cucumber Body Balm in my bathroom cupboard. The green tea ingredient is an extract listed near the bottom of more than a dozen of components—but that's not unusual for tea-infused beauty items.

Marriott Hotels: At Marriott Spas, guests can enjoy the impressive Thann bath product line (as I did do in Montréal, Quebec). The hand wash is derived from organic chamomile, sunflower seed, tea tree, orange, tangerine and nutmeg—ingredients that soften your skin. While I was 3,000 miles away from home, the hotel beauty items made me feel right at home, especially when I read the ingredient "chamomile."

Westin Hotels & Resorts: This luxury hotel offers a white tea-infused Heavenly Bath line, which includes shampoo, conditioner, body lotion, soap, and body wash. These products are available to purchase online so you can enjoy the tea-infused beauty and bath experience in the comfort of your home.

THE HERBAL TEA DIY BEAUTY RECIPES

When I logged on to the Internet in search of a pampering tea-infused spa treatment to book, I thought it would be an easy task, right? Wrong. A pure white tea and calming lavender Jacuzzi bath or soothing chai-ginger body massage while sipping a cuppa chamomile tea was my fantasy, complete with vanilla scented candles. I could see me there, all cozy and comfortable clad in a white plush robe. But it didn't happen like that. . . .

After the first hour of calling hotel spas around Lake Tahoe—a place where we do have high-end hotels with spas—I didn't find a Jacuzzi tea bath like the sessions I had experienced at a hotel spa in Reno. I was informed the spa closed and was being renovated until fall—no bubbly tea-infused water for me. During the second hour, I sipped a cup of chamomile blend tea (from Cal-a-Vie) to calm my frazzled nerves. (They do serve a wide array of teas but do not provide spa menu beauty treatments.) I was ready keep my appointment with a spa close to home. For almost 200 dollars, I could be wrapped up in a chai "cocoon" called a "body wrap"—but when the spa girl mentioned the word "claustrophobic" I cancelled. Images of Hannibal Lecter in protective gear haunted me.

Hours passed. Ready to forget a spa treatment I made a glass of iced black tea with orange slices and continued on my quest. I called a local Lake Tahoe nail salon that offered "green and peppermint manicures"; I recalled a past chocolate and strawberry infusion scrub before I had gotten a French manicure. "I can do a tea manicure!" I thought. Alas, I booked an appointment for my nails. I had proof: Tea does provide "brainpower" and stamina. I got another idea: "Why not purchase tea-infused beauty products (I found a white tea body and beauty line linked to a popular Westin hotel chain) and use them at home for spa day(s)," I thought. And I did just that. . . .

TEATIME PLEASURES IN THE HOME

As a tradition, I go out in the field for a *Healing Powers* series book day. But this time around, for tea, trying to find a spa with a beauty tea treatment menu, with baths, like the one I loved, was a feat I could not accomplish. I thought: "Wait. I have a pantry filled with black, white, green, red, and herbal teas. I have a new teapot, iced tea infuser, plenty of citrus, and ice cubes. Also, I have a freezer full of scones, biscotti, and Russian Tea Cookies (recipes are in chapter 20). What's more, I have tea-infused products—and I did order a few more: soap, body lotion. I can get spa'd at home."

On the morning of my spa day at home, I whisked my Australian Shepherd, Skyler, to the "spa"—aka kennel—to get a bath (it's challenging to rinse the soap out of his double coat) and a nail trim. Once the dog was gone, I went back home to pamper myself from head to toe.

HOME SWEET HOME

This spa day wasn't going to be like a super-structured Day-in-the-Life of a tea lover—it was more about relaxing and enjoying myself, something I forgot to do when working and taking care of the fur kids. I went to the shower—no dog, just the Siamese cat, Zen, and me. I lit lavender-scented candles. I turned on the shower until steam filled the room. My eyes met the massager tool I purchased; I was anticipating the pressure of water on my back, legs, and feet. I lathered my wet body with white tea body wash, washed my hair with a white tea shampoo and conditioner. I slipped into my soft and cozy gray robe (like the ones you can buy at luxury hotels) and matching slippers (a treat I purchased from Victoria's Secret after my last trip to the Hyatt Hotel—they offer robes fit for royalty in their grand bathrooms).

Into the kitchen to pour tap water into the steel tea kettle and wait for the sound of the whistle. I poured 2 cups of steaming hot water into the ceramic white teapot with a built-in strainer. I put 1 heaping teaspoon of white peony tea leaves in it and 1 heaping teaspoon of chamomile. I put biscotti that I made onto the saucer and was pleased with the presentation—one I created, one by one, from kettle to Italian cookie and a Russian Tea Cookies. After five minutes, I poured a cup and walked out onto the deck.

Back into the cabin, I made a tea bath (a tea concoction of herbal tea leaves, including calming chamomile and invigorating peppermint), and took the tub out onto the deck. Poured another cup of tea and sat outside again, dipped my feet (polish removed from my toes the night before) into the water. It was soothing and I awaited the tea infusion to do its magic before I dried off and gave myself a pedicure and polish with the new brown polish. My nails were next.

I was falling back into nature and looking up at the towering pine trees, and I realized no spa could give me what I had at home—peace and harmony in my own front yard. This DIY 90-minute session was bliss and nourished my body, mind, and spirit. No need to pay hundreds for a spa away from home. I'd been to Quebec and British Columbia, and stayed in pricey hotels with tea kettles, teas, and oversize marble soak tubs and spoiled myself with million-dollar views and room service. But my own spa time was perfect—and once dressed I was rejuvenated and ready to pick up my fresh pup, brush his clean coat, and take him for a walk. And, of course, treat myself to iced tea with fruit slices afterward. This day was a spa day, of sorts, to remember for days to come.

Here are some other DIY at-home recipes—using teas and tisanes—to try from head to toe that'll help you feel and look better.

Hair

In between visits to the hair salon? You can get highlights with tea. Blondes can try ½ cup brewed chamomile tea. Brunettes, use ½ cup strong black tea. Redheads, go for ½ cup red tea (red clover or rooibos).

Eyes

Puffy eyes can occur for a variety of reasons, whether it is lack of sleep or aging. Try black, green, white, or the classic chamomile tea bags. Put wet tea bags into freezer for about 10 minutes. Place one bag over each shut eye and chill for several minutes. If you prefer a quicker method, there are convenient eye wipes with tea extracts—less messy, more costly. You can find a variety of eye pads online. These ready-made pads can include tea extracts such as rooibos tea and green tea extract, depending on the brand.

Skin

Whether it's a tub or shower that you like, tea comes to the rescue. For shower lovers, go ahead and treat yourself to a soap or body lotion. (Tea-infused body and bath products are available online at major stores and beauty specialty shops.) If soaking in the tub is for you, try tying a couple of herbal tea bags around the water faucet. Any type will do but vanilla and citrus are relaxing and energizing.

Feet

You can create a tea footbath with your own choice of teas and tisanes or choose to use a basic soak concoction premade for you. I filled up a large plastic container of warm water and added the packet of the organic products. I soaked my feet for several minutes; the soles were rough from neglect, walking barefoot on the deck and ground, and chlorine from the swimming pool. The end result: Softer feet; however, I did massage each foot with coconut oil to heal crevices faster.

INSIDE A DAY IN THE LIFE OF A TEA LOVER

The following is a luxurious one-day spa plan to relax and renew your body and mind in the comfort of your home.

8:00 A.M. Wake up. Your day starts with an early morning walk outside with the dog. Then it's time for brewing a fresh cup of black tea. I recommend taking the tea back to bed (make sure the sheets are clean) and pretend you are at your favorite hotel. Sip your beverage.

8:30 A.M. Eat a tea-infused breakfast. Now it's time for a light and refreshing Tea Smoothie that's calcium-rich, quick and easy to prepare at home. (Recipe in chapter 2.) Pair your morning energetic smoothie with a homemade scone and Devonshire cream. (See chapter 20 for the recipes.)

9:00 A.M. Shower time. After breakfast, it's time to hit the shower like spa guests can do. Light scented candles. Use a tea-infused body soap, shampoo, and cream rinse. No rush. Take your time. Once done, use a large, fluffy towel, dry off. Step into a plush spa-like robe, slippers. But you've just begun.

9:30 A.M. Have a European tea facial. It's time for your facial. The following regimen is a spin-off from a spa that could be anywhere—but you are doing it yourself. Use tea-infused facial beauty products found online.

Begin with a cleanser. Then exfoliate the dead skin and rinse. Follow with a tea-infused facial massage (available for your skin—dry, oily, or normal). Lightly steam your face over a sink of hot water for several minutes. Pat dry.

11:00 A.M. Time to relax. Plan to spend the next hour listening to music or watching a cooking show on TV. No need to push yourself and work out or work. It's pampering time for you. What's more, how about taking a tea break? Brew yourself a cup of black or white tea. Sit down and savor the moment(s) for you.

12:00 P.M. Eat a Mediterranean-style lunch with tea flavor. You deserve a tea-licious lunch, so now it's time to treat your palate to a nutrient-dense meal that is low-fat, high protein, and easy to make at home (recipes in chapter 20).

1:00 P.M. Go swim. Getting a move on is part of the Mediterranean lifestyle. But no need to break a sweat and not enjoy your exercise. It's time to take dip and swim laps . . . but instead of fast freestyle why not try stretching-type swim strokes including breaststroke, sidestroke, and elementary backstroke? It will help calm you, and help you to burn off calories. After, treat yourself to a fruit juice mix with white or green tea (half-and-half).

2:00 P.M. Take a time-out. Now that your body is well fed and exercised, it's time to feed your mind. Go ahead—find your favorite relaxation room, sit down, and cozy up. Tune out intrusive thoughts or reverse it—problem-solve something that's been on your mind. After 20 or 30 minutes, you'll feel renewed and rejuvenated—lighter in mind, body, and spirit.

3:30 P.M. Snack time in the garden. Go to the freezer and take out a couple of tea cookies (see chapter 20). Tea time! Brew a cuppa like Brits do. No tea-bag time for you. Now is the time for a tea ritual: Pour water into the tea kettle and wait to hear the magical whistle. Put hot water into the ceramic teapot, rinse and pour the hot tea kettle water into it. Add a teaspoon of your favorite tea leaves and steep. Then, pour yourself a cup of tea to sip with your cookies. Go outdoors or sit by a window and look outside of your "tea garden" for the tranquility of it all.

4:00 P.M. Walk the dog or vacuum dog hairs. This is a perfect time to get moving again and you will be multitasking. Getting the canine companion its exercise and/or sucking up the fur will help keep both of you balanced and keep allergies at bay. Plus, each action is therapeutic. Note: If it is too cold or raining outdoors, hitting the treadmill (include the dog before or after) will suffice.

6:00 P.M. It's tea-infused dinnertime. You must be famished. It's time to enjoy a nutritious and satisfying meal that's tea-infused. Go to chapter 20 and take your pick of the savory dishes.

8:00 P.M. Give yourself a lavender bubble bath. When you finish dinner, it's time to top off your fun-filled tea day with a bath, or shower with calming lavender lotion or bubble bath. Fill a tub of water or turn on the shower (more inviting with a massage device and easy to install). Enjoy the warm sensations, savor the aromatherapy.

After the day and its events, it's time to put on lounge garb, cozy up on the couch or in your bed (clean sheets, please), and don't forget to bring yourself a cup of chamomile tea or an herbal blend of relaxing tea. Relax. It's been a beautiful day to remember and repeat as needed.

White and Green Tea Exfoliating Facial

This easy to make and easy to follow exfoliation recipe is mine and it works. The ingredients are most likely in your kitchen and ready to put to work. Go ahead and try it to reap the rewards of a do-it-yourself inexpensive beauty treatment that is priceless.

1 cup water
1 teaspoon green tea leaves, brewed
1 teaspoon white tea, brewed
2 tablespoons raw honey
1 teaspoon apple cider vinegar
1 teaspoon fresh lemon juice

Steep tea, green and white, in boiling water. In a small bowl, mix together honey, vinegar, and lemon juice. Remove tea from stovetop and mix in the other ingredients. Apply small amount of tea to your forehead, cheeks, chin, and neck. Leave on for 5 or 10 minutes. Rinse with cool water and pat dry with a clean towel. Follow with a moisturizer. Use this recipe twice a week for a rosy glow. The teas that are used in health spa beauty treatments can help guard your skin against the sun and air pollution. During this facial time, savor a cup of calming herbal tea.

Now that you've got the scoop on how to put tea beauty secrets to work for you, in chapter 17, it's time to discover how tea—all types—can help make your household, kids, and even pets happy and healthy. The people behind these innovations are thinking outside of the tea box, and it's time to embrace the amazing healing powers. These remedies using tea are connected to nature—a connectedness like honey and coffee. I've contacted some unforgettable people who respect the world of tea and future trends, as well as folks who put it all together so you and I can enjoy tea uses in all forms, types, and regions. What you're about to read will amaze you and leave you wondering: "Why didn't I do this before?"

TEA-CENTRIC HEALING HINTS TO STEEP

✓ Tea can help exfoliate, soften, and make your skin and hair look softer.

✓ Tea's antibacterial properties coupled with your skin's ability to hold in moisture can keep your skin hydrated, which makes it glow.

✓ Tea treatments include honey with natural plant extracts, essential oils, and other ingredients.

✓ White tea and green tea are often used in luxury health spa beauty treatments and store-bought beauty products. The tea can help to exfoliate, soften, and firm skin from head to toe to help both women and men look better and feel great, naturally.

✓ Tea masks, wraps, manicures, pedicures, baths, and much more are offered at health spas in America and around the world.

✓ But you don't have to go to a faraway pricey spa to enjoy tea-infused spa beauty treatments because they can be done in the comfort of your home.

Teamania: Trends to Household Hints

Where there's tea, there's hope.
—Sir Arthur Pinero

Once I was acclimated to Montréal, Quebec City was on journey's end since I didn't meet that goal in my twenties due to cultural shock. An early morning VIA Rail to the French-speaking town would take me to my final destination this time around—and black tea helped get me started. On the train I noticed my leather traveling bag had a scratch on it. I recalled tea can repair scratches on furniture, so why not leather? I dipped a napkin into the strong dark beverage three times. The liquid did indeed camouflage the imperfection *and* I felt alert for the four-and-a-half-hour train ride to the Promised Land—a place that promised European charm.

At Quebec City I entered a coffee and tea shop, run by younger people who spoke French and English. I ordered a Chai Latte. Not only did it make me feel at home but I also warmed up since it was chilly. I was ready to explore the streets—a horse-and-carriage tour to cobblestone streets of the old part of town. The chai—complete with black tea, spices, and steamed milk—boosted my sense of well-being and energy level, and thanks to the caffeine and the spices it was refreshing to drink.

21ST-CENTURY TEA INDUSTRY FACTS FYI

- Millennials, more so than older generations, are seeking innovation—teas that can give you an exotic vacation by the taste—and variety when it comes to current tea offerings—but baby boomers like novelty teas, too.

- Tea drinkers want to know more about origin, types of tea, tea garden names, flavor, description, etc., and tea shops and online vendors provide this to their customers.

- Food service continues to grow with tea becoming a more and more important offering in all types of restaurants.

- According to a forecast predicted by Packaged Facts, the food service tea market will likely have an edge in future growth as sales are expected to increase.

(*Source:* Tea Association of the U.S.A., Inc.)

THE SPLASH OF READY-TO-DRINK TEA

As I noted in chapter 1, tea in the form of loose leaves and tea bags are packed with more antioxidants than bottle tea. These RTD beverages, available in cans or bottles, attract tea lovers because of the convenience and allure of endless flavors. Companies are offering quality ready-to-drink teas (with natural ingredients, interesting tastes). This, in turn, may mean it's an avenue to offer more antioxidants like home-brewed tea.

One summer day I asked my sibling to pick up an RTD tea beverage for me—I was being adventurous and didn't dish a brand or flavor. (I did say "natural" though.) He picked out a large container of a nondescript brand tea. The nutrition label welcomed me with some good things, and not so good things: "No preservatives, sweetened with sugar." But I scrutinized the nutrition label and read: "Filtered water, sugar, tea concentrate, caramel color tea essence, and malic acid." Then, I read: "32 grams sugar and 38 milligrams sodium" per 12-ounce serving and 120 calories! It wasn't my cup of perfect tea (I would have selected a lemony-type tea with fun flavors, black tea and unsweet-ened).

So, I poured 4 ounces of ready to drink organic lemonade into a 16-ounce cup and filled up the rest with the RTD tea for the hot sum-mer's day. It was easy (no effort of brewing, straining, washing a kettle or teapot) and took me back to my Arnold Palmers with Dad. And, I was surprised at the clean taste of the ready-to-drink tea beverage. (Since then, I also brew my own black tea and add organic lemonade for the taste and health of it.)

The next day, I tried another brand: Snapple All-Natural Lemon Tea made from green and black tea; 16 ounces gives you 10 milligrams sodium, 150 calories, 36 grams of sugar, 42 milligrams of caffeine, fil-tered water, sugar, citric acid, tea, and natural flavors. The result: "Hello. My name is Cal. I am a part-time RTD fanatic. I love this stuff!" I prefer 8 ounces to cut the sugar, calories, and caffeine; and in-clude ready-to-drink teas (like this one) in my tea cupboard for busy and/or hot summer days or swimming days for the energy, tart taste, and convenience of not having to turn on a stove when it's 80 degrees or hotter.

The bottom line: RTD Teas are available in a variety of teas and fla-vors with or without lemon and sweeteners. These teas are available at major grocery stores, superstores, and convenient stores. Bottled bev-erages, like RTDs, can be tempting when you're on the go—a healthier pick than sugary sodas. But keep in mind they can include more sugar and fewer antioxidants than a homemade cup or glass of brewed tea, which give you control over what goes into it.

TEA FOR YOUR HOME—ROOM BY ROOM

Detox Your Kitchen

Clean up counters. Get fresh and sparkling countertops, whether it's marble or wood. Use a soft clean cloth soaked in a tea infusion (white tea or green tea) and wipe away dirt. Polish with a dry cloth until it shines. Not only will it be sparkling, the aroma will be fresh, too.

Wipe glass clean. Use brewed white or green tea mixed with water to get a clean surface.

Stamp out refrigerator stench. To remove bad odor from your fridge and freezer, try loose tea leaves. Place ¼ cup of flavored black tea leaves (such as vanilla or orange) in a small cup. It will suck up smells from fish to fowl and other scents.

Lighten up pantry cupboards. Instead of renovating the wooden rustic kitchen cupboards, I brewed a strong cup of lemon-scented black tea. I soaked a clean cloth with the liquid and wiped one cabinet after another. The wood felt clean and the chemical scent of commercial products was absent.

Wash the floors. Like wood cupboards using a black tea brew to clean grease and dirt off wood floors and even linoleum can work. Not only do the tannins get rid of the dirt and dust but if you buff it with a dry cloth after cleaning the surface you'll be greeted with a nice shine. A bonus: If you use a flavored black tea (like one with lemon or orange) the fragrance will linger and not be toxic like store-bought floor cleaners with chemicals.

Into the Living Room

Good-bye dust. Do you have dust bunnies on top of your wood furniture? Brew 1 cup of white or black tea. Pour the warm liquid into a clean spray bottle. Spritz the wooden dusty coffee table, chairs, and even leather (if it has been soiled). Clean with the grain, polish. I used this tea cleaning mix on weathered kitchen cabinets. Thanks to the antioxidants (tannins) the wood felt clean and there was a shine. Also, the scent was fragrant not intense like cleaners with chemicals, and the eco-friendly tea solution is safe for kids and pets.

Freshen up rugs. Instead of store-bought carpet cleaners, go green. Grind tea leaves (try green tea with citrus) in an herb grinder until powder. Shake and scatter the tea powder on areas that are dull or have an odor. Let it sit for several minutes, vacuum. Repeat if necessary. I tried using peppermint tea (loose leaf, I didn't grind it) on my oriental rug with a pet odor in the study. The first time, I didn't let it sit. No results. The second time around, I let it rest five minutes. It didn't work. The third time I ground a stronger and more fragrant blood orange tea, and let it sit for 30 minutes. As the adage goes, "the third time is a charm."

Wash windows. If your windows have dust, smears, and smudges, you don't have to use harsh window cleaners. Put 1 cup of brewed white tea with 1 cup of water into a clean plastic spray bottle. Spritz and wipe clean. Not only is it natural, you'll reap the reward of its antibacterial properties, too.

Personal Protection

Bathroom sink/toilet bowl. Using white tea leaves (ground fine) in the sink and/or toilet bowl can help to fade stains and it does act as a disinfectant, too. Let the tea sit for a few hours, rinse or flush. Repeat as needed.

Scent the air. The aroma of potpourri takes me back to the seventies and present-day shops like Pier 1 Imports with its fragrance that makes you feel energized and/or calm because of the inviting scent. You can duplicate this potpourri heaven by placing tea and tisanes in a small bowl. I used white tea leaves with notes of citrus and placed it on a high shelf in the bathroom.

Refresh drawers. To remove a musty smell or add a fresh scent to bathroom and bedroom drawers, put tea in nylon. I used favor gift pouch sachet bags with gold tone heart prints, in a sky blue color I found online. Use fragrant herbal tea leaves such as lavender or citrus.

Keep It Green Outdoors

Healthy up plants. What to do with used, wet tea leaves? Don't toss when you can feed those trees, bushes, and any greenery outside. Simply place tea leaves on the soil and lightly mix. (Do not use tea in your plants—indoors or outdoors—if you have a child, dog, or cat that digs in your greenery.)

Cool compost. If you have a compost bin, do toss your wet tea leaves in it because it will help expedite the breakdown and it's eco-friendly. Also, fragrant teas such as blood orange or peppermint may give it a nicer aroma upon opening the container.

Q&A: HAVE A CUPPA WITH A TEA MASTER

Who in the land of tea is a perfect companion to sit down with and chat it up about the topic of tea? Danielle Beaudette, a Certified Tea

Master. One of the first 15 individuals in the world to be certified as a tea specialist through the Specialty Tea Institute (STI), she has completed over 60 tea seminars at the World Tea Expo. She grew up in a French-Canadian family where tea was a staple in her home, although it was always "tea bag tea." Years later, the tide turned for this woman. Once smitten by her great aunt's tea collection, the software employee took an alternative route into Tea World, thanks to a meeting with Pamela Aaron, the "Texas Tea Queen." In a virtual interview, I asked Danielle about her world as a tea guru, its place in health and well-being for her and her business, The Cozy Tea Cart in Brookline, New Hampshire, which boasts a café complete with a chef.

Q: *Black or white? What is your favorite tea and why?*
A: By drinking one tea from each category of teas (white, green, oolong, black, and dark teas), I can enjoy the health benefits of each type of tea. But I would say I drink more black tea than any other tea. My daughters suffer from migraines, and starting the day with a few cups of black tea helps to ward off these headaches. (See chapter 15, "Home Remedies from Your Kitchen.")

I mostly drink straight tea that has not been blended with other herbs, spices, or flavorings. I thoroughly enjoy the taste of tea itself. However, I do enjoy the fruitier teas iced in the summer! Icing a fruity tea tends to bring out more of the fruity flavor, versus drinking it hot.

Q: *How has the tea industry changed for you from your fresh start to now?*
A: Tea consumers are asking more questions about their teas—about the countries of origin and the descriptions of the tea—they want to learn more about the healthy beverage they are consuming.

Q: *Chef Sabine Berke was trained in a European culinary school for five years and is constantly bringing new and exciting food to the menu. Please share about tea-infused eats and teas you've added.*
A: For some of our monthly formal afternoon teas, we serve Earl Grey Chocolate Truffles, Lavender Shortbread, Assam Tea–Infused Flourless Chocolate Torte, and Chai Scones. It is no secret that consuming the whole leaf is incredibly healthy for you.

Q: *While you are not a famous psychic eager to read tea leaves, you are savvy to tea and its workers in faraway lands. What changes do you foresee in the tea industry?*

A: For several years, when I have been in Asia, there has been talk about the average age of the tea plucker getting higher and the concern of how the leaves will be harvested once they are over the age limit to work. Their children are better educated and not following in the footsteps of their parents. This is a growing concern, and they are looking to new ways to harvest the tea leaves. Additionally, many of the countries have managed to control the wages so it is fair to the pluckers and factory workers. But there are ongoing labor issues in some countries that continue to need to be addressed.

Also, tea products will continue to appear on the market that aid in brewing and drinking the loose leaf tea more easily. The one thing that has probably held back some consumers of tea-bag tea is the misconception that whole leaf tea is a lot of work to brew. New and innovative products have been hitting the market to allow for ease in preparing the whole leaf tea such as loose tea travel mugs and stainless steel infusers for mugs. There are many more on the market and as these products develop, so will the demand for tea.

I have no doubt that the demand for good quality whole leaf tea will continue to grow in the coming years. With the information coming out of the scientific symposiums on tea every five years, we are gaining a wealth of knowledge on the health benefits of tea and are able to use that in promoting the whole leaf tea. As long as scientific research continues to occur, and continued education to the consumer takes place, the industry will continue to grow.

Q: *What teas do you carry that are big for tea lovers like me?*

A: Our signature blend, The Cozy Tea Cart Spice, is our biggest mover and definitely the flavored teas in all categories of tea. There are many teas available in our unflavored tea category. We try to get consumers to try straight teas or single estate teas (and create their own "special" blend, which we can re-create for them) to expand their palate into the world of tea. Like wines and scotches, they can find out what they truly like in these specialty teas.

THE FUTURE OF TEA

Certified Tea Master Daniel Johnson, The Cozy Tea Cart's Danielle, and I have all noticed that health awareness and health-care attitudes are shifting, whether you're a millennial or baby boomer or somewhere in between. Our actions are changing about how we eat, exercise, and take charge of our health instead of allowing the government to step in and tell us what is right and wrong.

"People are increasingly building their health, asking the right questions about food, and getting back to the earth. I feel part of our culture is returning to our roots. People are tired of an impersonal health-care system that urgently treats symptoms and does not support or rejuvenate the individual," explains Johnson.

As a health author for decades, I've been a follower of pairing holistic and conventional medicine but getting back to nature has been my focus. So when Johnson notes the messages we get through media and where we live and shop, such as "Get Fresh, Get Local," "Farm to Table," to exercise trends including mindfulness yoga—it's "opening people's eyes to the natural healing processes that are found in earth-based practices."

Welcome tea. "I feel as this trend continues people will be drawn to deepen their relationship with tea by learning its deeper practices and philosophies. Brewing tea slowly could transform the health of our country."

Indeed, life with tea is here to stay. Tea masters, medical researchers, nutritionists, and tea company producers agree that the tea industry is growing in America. As the author of books on coffee and chocolate, I see a similarity where tea tastes become more sophisticated and people want to try different teas and tisanes. Baby boomers are open to a variety of teas for healing powers and taste, while millennials ("echo" boomers) are adventurous when it comes to trying different teas from different regions for the thrill of it as well as health's sake. Elderly folks love their tea (often used to classics like black tea) while children will be introduced to more fruity herbal teas including rooibos. There is no definitive stereotyping to tea and tastes but generally speaking I sense my observations may be on target.

Also, while people around the globe are growing more aware of the health of their food (fruits, vegetables, dairy, and protein), being mindful of where your edibles come from and what's in them doesn't stop with tea.

Tea master Daniel Johnson is mindful of how man has played a role in the 21st-century tea industry. To find high quality, artisan tea is a challenge due to a variety of factors during the process to increase the production of tea leaves. "Our human footprint is deeply impacting our terroir," he says. "Pesticides, deforestation, and over-harvesting have damaged the topsoil of many growing regions." The creation of mechanized processed methods (CTC) to handle the increasing global demand for tea can affect the cup of tea you and I buy and drink. "Tea was once a simple leaf that was preserved for future enjoyment and nutritional value," he says. Nowadays, as with other superfoods, I believe we must question its source for good health and safety's sake. Enter the ideas at play—such as organic and fair trade, which include cocoa, coffee, chocolate . . . and tea.

GREEN LABELS, FROM GARDEN TO CUP

Here is an easy-to-understand lexicon for you to get and stay acquainted with the health of the tea industry and our planet, and what these terms linked to your cup of tea mean for you.

Biodynamic Farming	Farming conducted by following lunar cycles
Fair Trade	Fair market wages and prices, and ethical working producers
Bird-Friendly Tea	Tea grown so it doesn't bother the well-being of birds
Gluten-Free	Not containing gluten, a substance contained in cereal grains, especially wheat
Kosher	Tea meeting requirements of Jewish law, rabbi-certified
Organic	Tea leaves that haven't been sprayed with pesticides
GMO-Free	Non-genetically modified foods

Certified Rainforest Alliance	A non-governmental organization working to conserve tropical forests
Sustainable	A tea crop that doesn't harm people or the planet but preserves both
USDA Organic	United States Department of Agriculture accredited certifying agent verified tea product before labeled

HEALTHY TEA FENG SHUI TIPS

Welcome your home to the art of tea feng shui—the ancient Chinese art of placement—with a twist of tea and teaware. By putting stuff in the right spots in your kitchen, dining room, and outdoor deck or patio you can enhance the flow of positive "chi" or energy and avoid negative vibes, which may bring you good health and well-being. The ambiance of tearooms is light and airy, a place to relax and rejuvenate you and yours. Read on—you, too, can learn the art of tea feng shui for newbies, from room to room.

Declutter your teas. If you're a tea enthusiast, chances are you're going to have more than one box of tea bags in your pantry and a tea kettle. Rather than putting your tea stash all in one place, I advise storing your tea and teaware in different places for the feng shui of it all. You'll find tea tins and boxes (these have expiration dates) in my pantry, in canisters, and on a wall shelf. Also, these are sealed so I feel safe and secure that my fur kids won't get into the tea leaves or bags. I do not refrigerate or freeze tea (like I have done for coffee) but I do have some glass containers on the countertop (in a shaded area) with packaged tea bags. It's clutter-free, and it's a reminder that tea plays a role in my daily diet.

Flaunt tea tins. Some of the tin cans (such as ones from Harney & Sons) are so attractive and hold good memories of when I savored each and every tea that I couldn't toss them. Instead, once empty I put them in an assorted arrangement on a large wooden shelf. The collection is pretty and gives the kitchen a homey, rustic feel—chic and shabby.

Clean the tea kettle, teapot, tea leaf grinder. This is a task, but it's good energy to have a shiny steel tea kettle on the stovetop (an extra one above the kitchen island) or the hanging pots and pans rack. For the white ceramic pot after each use instead of dish soap (unless it's the eco-friendly tea-infused kind) use vinegar, water, and lemon (use hot water, let soak) and rinse. As far as the grinder goes, cleaning it after each use will keep it clean and you healthy.

Brighten up with lighting. In your kitchen (like tearooms), you'll be happier if it's airy and light, whether this is done by natural sun and/or the right lightbulbs. Fresh, light curtains or blinds will lighten up the room (do not close during the day) and your energy, so you'll want to brew a fresh pot of tea in the morning, afternoon, at dinner, or in the late evening.

Scent it up. Naturally, the aroma of tea, especially herbal teas, can give you scent-sational aromas for each season. Use a coffeepot and place one teaspoon of tea leaves in the coffee filter and brew a few cups of tea. (Go ahead—use your creativity and choose your fragrance. I recommend spice teas for autumn, chocolatey teas for winter, fruit teas for spring, and citrus teas for summer.)

Boost your mood with teacups, mugs, and glasses. Select your favorite teacups and place them together in a mug holder on the counter or install hooks inside the pantry door or above the top shelf. This is inviting for you or tea. Also, for tea glasses, line them up in rows in a furniture piece where you can see the inviting collection.

Use tea art. Framed tea prints can give your kitchen and dining room a cultural feel of the wide world of tea. You can go Mediterranean and follow the color theme of red, brown, and gold. Or decorate a room with a British ambiance with blue and white.

Pair tea mates. Set up glass canisters filled with homemade tea cookies or a tiered plate with muffins if you're expecting company. Not to forget a table runner, place mats, or a superb table cloth with cloth napkins.

Bring out the tea fruit, herbs, and spices. Tea—hot or iced—teamed with fresh slices of lemon, orange, or lime is inviting and healing. Also, whole sticks of cinnamon or sprigs of fresh mint are extra touches that can be added to many types of teas.

Hide the tea essentials. Teacups and saucers, stainless steel kettles and plastic tea pitchers, tablecloths or runners and place settings—they all can be beautiful and varied but having too many sets visible in your home will look cluttered unless you own a tearoom or are a tablescape diva. So choose your favorite teaware for an event or season and put away the rest.

Place tea books in piles. Books discussing tea topics such as baking, cooking, culture, and health can all be attractive and interesting for you and your guests. Arranging fascinating tea books in different rooms where tea is served can be attractive and timeless. Putting the cultural-type books in the living room, cookbooks in the kitchen, and health-related books in the dining room can all work well, especially when savoring a cup of tea.

A Bonus Tea Tip: Purchase a calendar with a tea time theme. It will keep you current on seasons and holidays—times when seasonal teas can up your tea game.

TEA LEAF READING, ANYONE?

Tearooms and specialty teas are among the tea trends growing in popularity within all age groups. During one of my trips to British Columbia, I visited Shangri-La Hotel Vancouver for a traditional afternoon tea. I ordered a pot of chamomile tea and the house apricot and currant scones. When the tea server clad in a cheongsam arrived at my table, I was intimidated. In hindsight, perhaps a high pour of the teapot (like the one Oliver does for show in the film *A Lot Like Love,* in the restaurant scene with Chinese flute music playing in the background) would have impressed her. She left the Blue Willow china teapot at my table. I didn't know *I* was supposed to strain the tea. Oops. Looking down at the wilted leaves in my cup, I sulked. I thought: "How can I drink this? The leaves will get stuck in my teeth." And the leaves steeped too long, so it was a dark yellow tea. When the server walked past my table, like a child I pointed to the flawed brew. (But at least I didn't pick up my saucer with the cup.) She replaced the full teacup with wilted tea leaves floating like dead goldfish. I felt my face warm up and turn red from embarrassment because I failed tea etiquette. I asked for a doggy bag for the pricey scones and walked out like a pup with its tail between its legs. I should have laughed at my gaffe and offered a tea leaf reading. But remember, I am a just a health author, not a tea master. What did I know?

Victoria Chocolate Mini Bundt Cakes with Lavender Honey Frosting

Chocolate is a must-have on a tea menu or in a tearoom. There are many recipes for chocolate cake but this one of mine seems to work on all levels. It is decadent, moist, and chocolaty, and serves up in perfect small portions. It can appease anyone at any age. Also, it's ideal for a birthday, Valentine's Day, or simply a sweet dessert for any time of the year.

2 cups cake flour
⅓ cup unsweetened premium cocoa powder
½ cup granulated sugar
½ cup light brown sugar
2 teaspoons baking powder
2 brown eggs
1 cup ricotta cheese
2 tablespoons sour cream
¼ cup European-style butter
1⅓ cup half-and-half
1 teaspoon pure vanilla extract
1 cup chocolate chips, 60 percent cacao

In a medium-size bowl, combine flour, cocoa powder, sugars, and baking powder. Then, add mixture of eggs, cheese, sour cream, melted butter, and half-and-half. Add vanilla and fold in chocolate chips. Pour batter into greased mini Bundt cake pan. Bake at 350 degrees for about 25 to 30 minutes. Cool.

LAVENDER AND HONEY FROSTING

2½ cups confectioners' sugar
4 tablespoons European-style butter, melted
1 teaspoon pure vanilla extract

1 teaspoon lavender leaves, ground fine into a powder (or strong brewed tea)
1 teaspoon honey
½ cup almond slices

In a bowl, mix sugar and melted butter to the consistency preferred. Add vanilla and lavender. Stir in honey. Spread with a knife on mini-cakes. Sprinkle with nuts and or sprinkles. Serves 20. Children love sprinkles.

Now that we've brought tea into baking and explained how to use it in a myriad of ways to make a happy home and maintain healthy kids, and taken a look at how the tea gods make this ingredient work wonders in everything from ready-made beauty products to do-it-yourself recipes—there's some unsettling news. Tea, although nature's infinite gift from 5,000 years ago, is not perfect and not for everyone for a variety of reasons. Go ahead, brew a cup of hot or iced tea, sit down and curl up to discover the downside of tea and how to get around some of the anti-tea challenges that you or yours may face.

TEA-CENTRIC HEALING HINTS TO STEEP

✓ While tea is known for countering common health ailments, it is also used for pets, kids, and household uses.
✓ Candles, furniture polish, and more are some of tea's versatile virtues.
✓ Tea furniture polish can clean your entire house.
✓ Tea-infused products, from candles to fun art, can be used by both kids and parents.
✓ Gardening tools, golf clubs, and leather goods are all things that can benefit from tea, an all-purpose cleaner and preserver of goods.

Not Everyone's Cup of Tea

*The morning cup of coffee has exhilaration
about it which the cheering influence of the
afternoon or evening cup of tea cannot be
expected to reproduce.*
—Oliver Wendell Holmes, Sr.

During my trip to Eastern Canada both tea and tisanes were part of my diet regime, from the fast-paced industrious city of Montréal to French-speaking Quebec City, a place of European Old-World charm. I cannot imagine a world without tea. At 3:30 A.M. on the day I was scheduled to travel to the Montréal-Pierre Elliott Trudeau International Airport, the hotel rang my room. I struggled to get up, pack, and bathe. I could have brewed a cup of joe but I didn't want the strong caffeine jolt so early in the morning. Thus, I made a cup of green tea. In the tub, it gave me the perfect balance of energy and brainpower to get my bags in order, check out of the hotel, hail a cab, and go through customs . . . nothing as challenging as when I arrived in Quebec after 3,000 miles. I was blindsided by a young customs agent woman who grilled me, the Northern California woman clad in jeans, a sweater, minimal makeup, and long locks. I craved a cup of strong chamomile tea to stay calm through the one-hour interrogation as to why a single woman would travel to Canada, which gave me memories of decades ago when I was kept at the border with my dog—and had no ID. I sat cross-legged on the floor—both times—tea-less. I had come full circle but didn't have a canine companion for moral support—just fantasies of tea waiting for me in the hotel room I had booked. As noted in chapter 16, I got my wish.

Once in my hotel room a cup of hot chamomile put me to sleep like in the Peter Rabbit tale. Tea and tisanes have their special time and place whether you are home or away because of their multitude of benefits, including flavor and aroma, and how they affect your mind and body. But savoring a cup of tea isn't always a simple choice. . . .

Is tea for everyone? It's not. There are many reasons why drinking tea doesn't work for people, including the side effects of herbal non-teas, and, of course, taste. Let me take you through the ins and outs of the world of tea and show you why specific types may not be your cup of tea—and what to do about it.

CAFFEINE WITH YOUR TEA?

Tea, like other superfoods such as coffee, is good for you in moderation but anything with caffeine when consumed in excess can have some not-so-great side effects. "Although the caffeine content of tea varies," says dietitian Vandana Sheth, "if you are extremely sensitive to caffeine, it may increase your anxiety level." Take a look at the caffeine intake you'll consume in a cup of tea and make your decision which type is right for you at the right time.

CAFFEINE CONTENT OF TEA TYPES

Tea/Non-Tea	Caffeine	Serving Size
Black tea	70 milligrams	8 ounces
Green tea	20 milligrams	8 ounces
Herbal tea	0 milligrams	8 ounces
Oolong tea	45 milligrams	8 ounces
Red tea	0 milligrams	8 ounces
White tea	15 milligrams	8 ounces

Health authorities will tell you 400 milligrams per day is the safe amount of caffeine for most healthy adults. If you do not want too much caffeinated tea, knowing green tea and white tea contain less caffeine than black tea and oolong tea gives you choices. But it doesn't stop there. Herbal teas are caffeine-free and often are ideal if it's late in the afternoon or nighttime and you don't want to get energized mentally or physically.

But note: While decaffeinated teas are available and these tisanes sometimes lack taste, some tea companies have perfected the flavor of decaf teas. Not unlike decaf coffee, the decaffeinated tea process removes caffeine (but not 100 percent) and preserves a lot of the flavonoids. This, in turn, means you can still get a good amount of healthy catechins in a cup of decaf tea for your heart's sake, according to studies.

It's not just the caffeine in tea that can make it not your cup of tea, but there are other reasons why you may want to switch your brew from tea to tisane or tisane to tea or use it in a different way, whether it is topically or for your household. Speaking of the home, enter children.

HERBAL TEAS FOR KIDS—YOU BET!

Teas with caffeine are not advised for children, but besides herbal teas, another trend that is popular around the world is bubble tea, also tagged boba or pearl tea. I first noticed the item on a tearoom menu (in the children's category) at the Vancouver, British Columbia Fairmont Hotel. But later after doing my homework it was evident that this special tea goes back decades. . . .

Specialty tea experts will share the tale that in the late 20th century in Taichung, Taiwan, Lin Hsiu Hui got a brainstorm while working at the Chun Shui Tang Teahouse. When eating a tapioca pudding (the dessert I grew up on in the sixties), she put a bit of it into her iced tea beverage. The odd gesture ended up being a popular trend especially for children in the other teahouses in Taiwan . . . and the tea was called bubble tea. It is a cold blended beverage in a variety of flavors with "pearls" of tapioca on the bottom of the beverage, which are slurped through a straw. Bubble tea is served in tearooms and available online at specialty tea shops. Health Check: Serve in moderation. Do not overindulge because of the high sugar content, which health authorities believe can trigger obesity and other health problems.

Pot of Tea

❖ ❖ ❖

2 cups fresh tap water
2 teaspoons bubble tea

Pour water into a tea kettle. When water is near a boil or the kettle whistles, remove. Pour water into a pot with a diffuser. Place tea in it. Steep for 3–4 minutes. Serves 2.

TEAS ARE NOT ONE CUP FIT FOR ALL

Certified Tea Master Daniel Johnson knows as I do that teas and tisanes come with a myriad of healing powers—and some come with side effects. "It is important to note that not all teas are good for everyone," he notes. "If you have a sensitive stomach the bitter and cold, antioxidant-loaded green tea may cause you distress. You would most likely find more health benefit and enjoyment from a fully oxidized black tea," adds the tea guru. That said, since our bodies differ in what we need, whether it is white tea or black tea or a tisane, it's a blessing that tea is versatile. "Tea gives us a gift by possessing many forms," says Johnson who adds, "the greatest health benefits of tea are drawn from using the most appropriate tea for each person."

GREEN TEA AND RADIATION: IS IT SAFE?

On March 11, 2011, a Japanese earthquake and tsunami happened, as well as the Fukushima nuclear disaster. Nuclear reactors affected regions of Japan, and its tea industry was also hit. The fact is, parts of Japan and even the West Coast have been disturbed by the disaster. And the green tea industry is not immune to the fallout.

Consumers of green tea and matcha are concerned about its quality; I, a health-conscious tea lover in California who asks the butcher

"Where does this fish come from?" and drinks bottled water because the arsenic in Lake Tahoe groundwater is questionable, am among those concerned. When I received an order of matcha powder, for example, it was a sobering experience to open the package and read a notice informing me that the contents had been checked for radiation exposure. On Day One, I moved the container from the kitchen to the study's file cabinet. Then, I called a few friends and asked: "What would you do?" I tossed it. Later, I went online thinking, "I'll buy my green tea from China." I discovered green tea from China is dealing with lead issues.

Meanwhile, articles on green tea and radiation are less frightening years later after the disaster—but concern about the safety of green tea from Japan is not off the table. "Is it Safe to Drink Green Tea from Japan?" greeted me in seconds when I did an online search on the topic. Tea proponents tell me different things. Some say to relax; others caution and say be mindful and trust your source. A few tea companies tell me their green tea is nowhere near the epicenter of the great earthquake or nuclear meltdown; and tea gurus tell me all the tea in Japan is checked and no worries. But I still am a bit cautious as a tea lover and health author.

Tea master Daniel Johnson says, "If purchasing Japanese teas, learn where it's grown. Certain regions have not been impacted by radiation and continue to produce very healthy, high-quality tea." He adds that we should become informed tea consumers, and to learn to trust our supplier. "They should be comfortable answering any questions about the growing location and possible contamination of any of their teas." My final word: Many consumers may choose to avoid Japanese tea products considered safe by the government. Others will get a sense of safety from the merchant and use the tea in moderation.

HOLD THE TEA . . . IT'S TOO HOT!

The word is, the World Health Organization claims hot drinks like tea and coffee are a "probable" cancer trigger. As the reports go, the group's International Agency for Research on Cancer (IARC) looked at about 1,000 studies that investigated a link between high-temperature drinks and cancer. The findings: Drinking very hot beverages—anything above 149 F—is linked to a higher risk of developing cancer of the esophagus. The results were published in *The Lancet Oncology*. So, it's time to be mindful, and let your cup of hot tea cool before you sip and savor the healthful brew.[1]

KOMBUCHA: IT'S HOT, BUT . . .

Like any food or tea, some types are not 100 percent perfect for 100 percent of people. Kombucha, the fermented tea discussed earlier, may not be your cup of tea despite its healing powers. Yes, there are plenty of warnings (like other teas) to consider before drinking this tea.

If you have a weakened immune system or other serious health conditions, it is advised to consult with your health-care practitioner before trying a probiotic like kombucha. And pregnant women who have never consumed probiotics are generally advised against starting them during pregnancy.

CAN TEA STAIN YOUR TEETH?

Truth be told, when I accepted this long-awaited book project, coping with teeth stains from trying new tea did cross my mind. "What about my teeth?" I pondered. After all, as a baby boomer I have treated my pearly whites with tender loving care and have faced some challenges: braces, fillings, a few crowns, a bonding, and regular dental checkups.

I'm hardly alone. Some folks are turning away from black tea and drinking green tea and fruit teas to stave off the off-color tea stains *and* caffeine. But note as I did, fruit teas are acidic (not unlike lemonade, orange juice, and vinegar) and are not tooth-friendly for tooth enamel. Also, like coffee, tea contains tannins—which *can* discolor teeth to shades of gray and yellow.

But there are some easy, practical tips to use to minimize tea and teeth stains. Use a straw when drinking tea—any variety—and the liquid will not affect your teeth as much. Also, after a cuppa, rinse with water and brush soon after. Using a gentle, less abrasive whitening toothpaste, a soft toothbrush, and brush at a 45-degree angle. Regular dental cleanings and polishings can help lessen stains caused by tea and other good-for-you Mediterranean diet foods, including berries and wines. Also, a professional teeth-whitening procedure does indeed work and can help you achieve and enjoy a whiter shade for your pearly whites. So if you are mindful about regular dental care, you can have your tea and drink it, too.

White Tea Eggnog

❖ ❖ ❖

Eggnog is a rich beverage that captivates people in autumn, winter, and through the holidays. You can healthy up that cup of eggnog, too, by using a premium, low-fat brand, adding tea and spices. Can you spell tea-licious?

2–4 cups white tea (Harney & Sons White Vanilla
    Grapefruit, tea sachets)
2 cups gourmet premium low-fat eggnog (Horizon
    Organic)
Fresh ground nutmeg, to taste
Cinnamon sticks (garnish)

In a saucepan, combine tea and eggnog. Stir over medium heat until mixture is hot but not boiling. Top with nutmeg. Garnish with cinnamon sticks. Serves 4–6.

To recap, if you have a sensitivity to a certain tea due to caffeine or sugar (if it's a ready-to-drink tea), there are options, whether it is going decaf, unsweetened, or switching to another type of tea or tisane. And using tea topically—for health and beauty—is another way to get your tea.

In the future, I sense that tea—black, white, and green—will be used more in kitchens and households as well as medical clinics and hospitals around the globe. In chapter 19, "The Joy of Cooking with Tea," you'll be amazed at how versatile teas and tisanes are in cooking and baking—and wonder, "How did I ever cook up a dish without this superfood?" And your life in the kitchen as you know it will change.

TEA-CENTRIC HEALING HINTS TO STEEP

✓ There is a wide variety of teas and tisanes, so if one is not your cup of tea, no need to worry.

✓ Options to switch to another tea or tisane are readily available if you do your homework, consult with your health practitioner, and keep an open mind.

✓ Tea with caffeine should never be given to infants, toddlers, or tweens due to its potential negative effects.

✓ But many herbal teas may be fine for children and definitely a better beverage choice than sugary sodas or caffeine-fueled energy drinks!

✓ Further scientific research is needed in the United States and around the world to prove that teas can help heal a variety of health ailments and diseases.

✓ Tea is not a cure-all for every ailment and disease and hype about its healing powers needs to be brought down to earth. But tea is a gift . . .

✓ Tea used solo and paired with a nutrient-rich diet can often be a godsend to people (of all ages) in a variety of ways.

PART 8

TEA RECIPES

The Joy of Cooking with Tea

*You can never get a cup of tea large enough or
a book long enough to suit me.*
—C. S. Lewis

One early fall at Lake Tahoe I packed my bags, and flew to British Columbia to attend the Canadian Coffee & Tea Show for the thrill of it. After classes on tea, I was revitalized (blame it on the tea cupping) and made rounds to Stanley Aquarium and tearooms for relaxation and amusement.

At my visit to the past place called The Urban Tea Merchant I was greeted by a savvy tea master/server. While admiring the choices on the tea menu, I chose my tea and treat. It was the Sommelier's Tea Suggestion: Dragon Gate Tea: a blend of white, green, and oolong teas with "lusty tonalities of ginger and a hint of sweet mint and citrus" paired with a small scoop of tea-infused crème caramel ice cream. This tea lover's treat left me wanting more but isn't that the idea rather than overindulging in dessert?

In a foreign country all alone I felt a sense of security when sipping the tea and enjoying the taste of the ice cream. Was it my first time enjoying a food with tea in it? The answer is no. I thought back to my book *The Healing Powers of Honey*. Recipes like Honey Tea Bread made with a strong brew and Asian Shrimp with orange pekoe tea were two dishes that came to mind as I sipped a second cuppa from the pot of tea.

As I look back at that afternoon, my face turns a shade of red. I asked my server if I could interview the founder—Mr. Twining. I was clueless about the roots of the man behind the history of tea—and my ignorance was no doubt obvious.

The experience was pleasurable with the multiplicity of British Columbia's London-Asian vibe, but the south shore of Lake Tahoe was on my mind and in my heart. The thing is, while enjoying a cup of tea and ice cream—both comforts delights to me—it made me feel comfort, like I do at home; a lifeline to my Old Tahoe–style cabin nestled in pine trees. While I was feeling waves of homesickness amid a place I love to be, it was a powerful moment of a season of contentment, because I knew it was a special afternoon and tried to savor it, every minute—a time to put my lonely feelings aside while enjoying tea time *and* the place I was supposed to be.

That evening, I was due to pay a visit at the Fairmont Hotel Vancouver for high tea . . . another experience to treasure. I ordered white tea and was served a pot and teacup—not a tin kettle like you get at coffee shops. Not a big dinner person, I ordered the house Notch8 Restaurant + Bar dinner salad (organic leaves, heirloom vegetables, pomegranate & roasted shallot vinaigrette), signature bread (stout, comte cheese, mustard seed), and a stack of julienne fries. I did not have a tea-infused edible but the Fairmont white tea selection was perfect.

These recipes, more than 30 tea-licious rustic recipes, are full of Mediterranean diet food including fruits, vegetables, fish, poultry, whole grains, herbs, spices, and plenty of water for teas and tisanes. The dishes provided by chefs, tea masters, tea enthusiasts, and me contain a variety of teas—black, white, green, and herbal teas. Plus, superfoods such as healthful chocolate, honey (often paired with tea and non-teas), and olive oil and vinegar are part of many of the recipes, too.

Putting tea to work in recipes is not a secret to spa or celeb chefs. Seasoned chefs know by experience and creativity that teas—all types—can and do add flavor and aroma in a variety of ways to entrees and desserts. Not only does tea boast antioxidants, and contain no calories or sodium, but tea-infused dishes are fun to make because of the end results. Tea's versatile ways to flavor up everything from bread, fish, and fowl to pastries and chocolate continue to please the palate.

For best results, use the tea and tisane type mentioned in each recipe. However, feel free to use your own brand and form (tea bags, leaves, or powder). Before you get started and dip into cooking and baking with tea, I want you to first take a peek at some cooking-with-tea tips.

TEA-LICIOUS TIPS FOR TEA CUISINE

Tea	Flavor	Uses
Black	Strong, bold taste	Poaching egg, glazes for fish, poultry meats
Fruit	Floral, sweet, fruity	Cakes, cookies, muffins, smoothies, vinaigrettes
Green	Grassy, distinct	Crepes, fish (trout, tuna), pasta, sauces, soups
Herbal	Spicy, earthy	Breads, cakes, cookies, glazes, and marinades for lean meats
Chamomile	Mild	Rice
Jasmine	Mild	Rice
Matcha	Grassy, distinct	Cakes, cookies, ice cream, smoothies
Pu-erh	Strong, earthy	Poultry, stir-fry dishes
Rooibos	Sweet	Chocolate (any type) mousse
White	Mild	Sauces for fish, iced tea cocktails, poached salmon, sorbet, soups

(*Source:* Based on recipes in this book.)

STORING TEA TIPS FOR TEA ENTHUSIASTS

Finding and acquiring quality tea is an art. Once you have tea (leaves and bags) that you're proud enough to show off to family and friends (like one does with a fine wine or olive oil collection), it's time to store tea the way that will preserve it as long as possible. During my journey in Coffee and Chocolate Worlds, I discovered that there is an ongoing debate amongst experts about the proper way to keep your beans and truffles fresh. And it's not much different when I dish the topic with tea people.

Keeping your tea—leaves and bags—in a dark, cool pantry is the way you're told to do it. It seems to me that storing tea is like storing treasured coffee—but not exactly. When I was gifted coffee—pounds and pounds of beans—there is no way I felt good about stashing it in my pantry. "What if there is an earthquake in the Golden State?" I pondered. My dog or cat could get into the not pet-friendly beans and pet game over. So I did (and still do) put airtight bags of coffee beans in both the refrigerator and freezer. But tea is different. . . .

Unopened small tea boxes and tea cans are lined up on shelves in my dark pantry. Some of these teas go back one year—but when I open each one as I use it, they are fine. However, I admit I feel more secure using the teas that have an expiration date on the container—and many do indeed. In fact, some of the dates go beyond one year.

You can be the final judge (there is no tea police) on how to store your favorite teas to keep them at their best for the freshest pot of brew. But here are a few tips just in case you're open to more tea safe-keeping despite tea having a fairly long shelf life.

- Freezing is not great for tea leaves.

- The best way to store your tea bags and tin cans is to keep them sealed.

- Do not allow your tea to be exposed to sunlight or moisture.

- Better to buy smaller batches of tea that you can use in a few months, rather than big batches that will not be as fresh.

- If the tea container does not have an expiration date, write down the date of purchase when you bring it home.

IT'S HEALTHY TEA BREWING TIME

Ever wonder what water temperature is ideal for an ideal cup of tea? If you scrutinize different charts created by tea companies and often noted on their tea packages, it may daze and confuse you since the time and brewing temperature may differ.

The less oxidized a tea is, the cooler the water temperature and shorter steep. Use filtered water for best results. Simply follow these numbers *and* your taste buds as a guide—you are enjoying tea for flavor and health benefits. Also, for best results, follow the instructions on the tea brand label. Health Check: And note, don't forget to let a steaming cup of tea cool before you sip!

Here is a more comprehensive steeping baseline (including heat) for you to follow that will preserve those healthy antioxidants in your tea (bag or loose leaf). But note, different brands vary with their guidelines.

Tea	Serving Size	Water Temperature	Steeping Time
Black	1 tsp./8 ounces	212° Fahrenheit	3 minutes
Green	1 tsp./8 ounces	180° Fahrenheit	2 minutes
Oolong	1 tsp./8 ounces	195° Fahrenheit	3 minutes
White	1 tsp./8 ounces	180° Fahrenheit	3 minutes
Herbal	1 tsp./8 ounces	205° Fahrenheit	3–4 minutes

SEASONAL TEAS AND FOUR SEASONS

Tea companies and tea masters will tell you that in the 21st century the selection of teas and tisanes is forever expanding and attracting tea lovers. New, improved varieties continue to attract people into the vast land of teas—often custom-tailored for the four seasons. Blends of specialty organic teas from a variety of countries including China and Sri Lanka attract. Scented and flavored teas including pumpkin spice for autumn and peppermint bark through the holiday season are in demand in homes, like mine, and at coffee and tea shops. And scented and flavored white tea and black tea with notes of florals, herbs, and fruits are favorites in the summertime as iced teas.

Winter

It's the Season: 'Tis the season of colder days, longer nights. It's a time when wildlife hibernates, the first snowfall arrives, firewood is stacked, and the heater kicks on. A cup of hot black tea for energy in the morning and afternoon is perfect paired with tea cookies infused with Earl Grey or lavender.

Healing Seasonal Teas: Dark and black teas and chai are ideal for wintertime. Holiday spice tea such as black Ceylon tea with notes of orange and cinnamon, as well as herbal teas including chamomile to help keep calm during hectic holidays and rooibos blends are popular through Valentine's Day.

Superfoods with Tea: cabbage, chia seeds, citrus fruits, and pears

Spring

It's the Season: Once winter days are almost over, it's time for renewal and to make your home and body lighter for warmer days ahead. It's common for me to brew a pot of white tea in the afternoon and a chamomile flower blend at night to welcome sleep during the Daylight Savings Time change. Healthful sandwiches paired with teas, vegetarian entrees, and green salads with tea-infused dressings come into play. It's time to shed extra unwanted winter weight, and get a move on with lighter fare.

Healing Seasonal Teas: Detoxifying green tea and citrus tea (hot or iced) are popular during this time of lightening up. Organic spring jasmine, chamomile citrus, organic white peony, and rooibos blends are superb springtime teas that are perfect for the season of fresh beginnings.

Superfoods with Tea: apricots, artichokes, carrots, and spinach

Summer

It's the Season: Summer is a time to get a light touch and change of linens, clothes, opened screen windows, and fresh air. It's the time I relax in the morning with a cup of flavored black tea (for the caffeine boost) so I can get more physical and be more active in the longer days and nights of summertime. Iced tea makes a splash during this season of sun and frolic. Brewing black tea and infusing it with fresh citrus including limes, oranges, and lemons, in a pitcher filled with ice is a must-have. Pairing a glass of iced tea with summer fruit mini scones or cucumber tea sandwiches and fresh vegetable and fresh fruit salads and grilled fish is ideal.

Healing Seasonal Teas: Fruit teas (such as blackberry and strawberry), white peony with fruit notes, and iced black tea are summer favorites to help the body cool down and feel energized. Other fruity profiles including blood orange, citrus hibiscus herbal, mango black, and peach fruit teas are ideal for the summertime.

Superfoods with Tea: blueberries, peaches, pineapple, and tomatoes

Fall

It's the Season: In the Sierra at Lake Tahoe and other regions around the United States and globe, there are hints of autumn, whether it is the transformation in hues of tree leaves or a crisp chill in the air. Tea is a joy during this new season. I love to sip a cup of cinnamon or any spice tea paired with a fresh, warm mini vanilla scone either homemade or purchased at a coffee shop in Seattle—fall is the time I seem to visit.

Healing Seasonal Teas: Pumpkin spice tea, peppermint bark, chocolate spice, and gingerbread teas are in demand, as well as green tea and green tea blends—flu and cold-fighting powers are always welcome during the autumn harvest. Not to ignore warming chai with its black tea and spices and Earl Grey, a black tea with orange peel and oil of bergamot.

Superfoods with Tea: apples, grapefruit, pumpkin, and sweet potatoes

THE TEA HEALTH-BOOSTING FIVE-DAY MENU PLAN

This diet plan is a sample of what you can create day by day with the help of teas and tisanes. Refer to the chapter on the Mediterranean diet to see the balance of food groups. This five-day tea diet plan is based on the seasons and nutritious whole, clean foods that are healthier than processed fare.

Recipes* can be found in previous chapters, especially at the end of each chapter, or in this Tea Menu chapter. You can mix and match to suit your personal taste and custom-tailor it to the season.

Day 1: Winter

Breakfast:
1 Raisin Scone* with Devonshire cream & honey
1 cup fresh-squeezed orange juice
1 Pot of Tea for Two (English Breakfast Tea)

Lunch:
1 Tea Sandwich (Organic Egg Salad*)

Snack:
Sweet Tea*
Russian Tea Cakes*

Dinner:
Pork Tenderloin with Tea*
1 serving Orange Squeeze Tea Spiced Carrots*
1 garden green salad with warm cruciferous vegetables

Snack:
Mug of Tea (Chamomile)
1 cup fresh fruit

Day 2: Spring

Breakfast:
1 cup honey Greek yogurt with ½ cup fresh fruit
1 Chai Pumpkin Seed Muffin*
Pot of Tea for Two (Black Tea)

Lunch:
1 serving White Tea Spring Rolls*
1 serving green vegetable

Snack:
1 fresh fruit
1 cup of white citrus tea

Dinner:
> 1 serving chicken with citrus tea rub
> 1 serving potato
> 1 serving green salad with fresh spring vegetables

Snack:
> 1 mini scone
> Mug of Tea (green or herbal)

Day 3: Summer

Breakfast:
> 1 homemade buttermilk waffle served with honey or syrup
> 1 bowl fresh fruit
> Pot of Tea for Two (Black Tea)

Lunch:
> Tea Sandwich (Cold Tuna, Cracked Wheat Bread)*
> Iced Tea infused with slices of orange, lemon, and lime

Snack:
> 1 serving whole grain chips and salsa
> 1 cup of tea

Dinner:
> 1 serving Scallops in Black Tea*
> 1 serving green salad with summer vegetables

Snack:
> 1 slice Pretty Plum Earl Grey–Infused Tart*
> 1 Mug of Decaffeinated Flavored Black Tea

Day 4: Fall

Breakfast:
> White Tea and Strawberry Smoothie*
> 1 cup chai

Lunch:
Tea-Infused Mushroom Soup*
Tea Sandwich (Grilled Cheese)
1 Mug of Tea (Pumpkin Spice)

Snack:
Pot of Tea for Two
1 serving Biscuits* and honey

Dinner:
1 large serving Organic Baby Spinach with Organic Tea Seed Oil
    Dressing*
Baguette with real European-style butter

Snack:
1 slice Apple Chamomile Tea Cake*
Mug of Spice Tea (Cinnamon)

Day 5: Year-Round

Breakfast:
1 serving Chia Seed Porridge and Pot of Tea for Two*

Lunch:
Tea Sandwich (Peanut Butter & Jelly*)
1 serving vegetables

Snack:
Mug of Tea (White Tea)
1 serving tea-infused ice cream

Dinner:
1 serving black tea-infused brown rice
1 serving cruciferous vegetables, sautéed in garlic, olive oil, and
    butter
Pot of Tea for Two (Green Tea)

Snack:
1 fortune cookie
Mug of Herbal Tea (Chamomile)

A healthful breakfast is a perfect way to begin the day as spa-goers do at renowned resorts around the world. Porridge with healing super-foods, including chia seeds, almond milk, honey, fruit, spices, and a cup of hot tea is a way to warm you up and give you an energizing jump start.

Chia Seed Porridge and Chai

¼ cup chia seeds
1 cup almond milk (or coconut milk)
½ banana, mashed
½ teaspoon vanilla extract
½ teaspoon honey

TOPPING

1 cup pecans, toasted
¼ cup cranberries, soaked in water 10–30 minutes to hydrate (Author's Note: I soaked the cranberries in herbal lemon-flavored tea (Bigelow).)
1 teaspoon cinnamon

Soak chia seeds, almond or coconut milk, banana, vanilla extract, and honey for two-plus hours in the refrigerator. Add pecans, berries, and cinnamon before serving. Serve chilled.

(*Courtesy:* Cal-a-Vie Health Spa)

Good Morning, Chocolate Chai Tea!

❖ ❖ ❖

1 cup water
½ cup organic 2% chocolate milk
1½ teaspoons chai (loose leaves)
Honey to taste (optional)
1 dollop whipped cream
Cinnamon to taste

In a small pan, combine water and milk and warm on medium heat until hot but not boiling. Add chai and honey (if preferred sweeter). Reduce heat to low for a few minutes. Strain into cup. Top with whipped cream and a dash of cinnamon. Serves one.

You are going to enjoy the last chapter—recipes for you to create and use for your own tea menu at home. Tearooms are a wonderful place that invite you to feel calm, energized and rejuvenated, and pampered—an ultimate escape. In the "Tea Menu" chapter I categorized recipes in a format similar to a tea menu for your pleasure.

TEA-CENTRIC HEALING HINTS TO STEEP

✓ Cooking with tea is fun and can make your recipes more flavorful, especially if you learn how to pair the right teas and tisanes with the right foods.

✓ Storing tea (loose leaf to bags and sachets) must be done properly or you'll not have a fresh pot or cup of tea. Expiration dates are great but so is putting your teas and tisanes in the proper place.

✓ Brewing temperature and time for steeping can vary. It's best to follow the guidelines from your tea brand and basic rules noted in this chapter.

✓ Seasons and teas are important. Savoring seasonal teas will make your tea drinking much more enjoyable and you'll be able to feel the season.

Tea Menu

*To a philosopher all news, as it is called, is gossip,
and they who edit and read it are old women over
their tea.*
—Henry David Thoreau

When I entered my first but not last tearoom in Vancouver, British Columbia, it took me back to my first tea party. Remember, I was the kid with a big imagination from the suburbs, the one who threw a tea party with imaginary tea, animal crackers, and stuffed animal friends. I was the little girl who grew up and sensed there was a big tea world to explore—and did just that. So imagine how my heart skipped a beat (think Edgar Allan Poe's "The Tell-Tale Heart") and the unforgettable serene environment took my breath away.

As I walked into the Tea at the Top on the 15th floor at the Fairmont Hotel Vancouver it had me at first sight. I was wooed by the ambiance of a light and airy room as well as chatting with my gracious server. I was treated to a pot of hot tea, house-made warm butter and raisin scones (dog-ear the recipe at the end of chapter 1), and honey yogurt panna cotta with macerated fruit. It was a comforting home away from home that took me to a place I love and a place I wanted to be.

Tearooms and gardens are a place for everyone but if you can't whisk away on a plane or by car ride to tea utopia, you can create your own tearoom in the comfort of your home. My tea menu—a creation from many tearooms I've visited—is something that'll make you smile each time you create a dish and serve it to you and yours. Bon appetit!

THE HEALING POWERS SPECIAL TEA MENU

Biscotti, Croissants, Muffins, Scones

Sweet pastries with a European twist are sweet to the eye and palate for breakfast, lunch, afternoon tea, or high tea. A pot, mug, cup, or glass of tea—hot or iced—and a pastry paired with clotted cream or tea-infused jam is the way tea lovers love their cuppa, whether it's in Asia, England, France, or the United States. Tea—all types—and pastries are a perfect marriage. Chocolate biscotti and green tea is a match made in tea heaven. A buttery plain croissant with a strong cup of Earl Grey can't be beat. A bran muffin with an iced White Peony or a blueberry scone with a cup of chai can convert a coffee lover to a tea enthusiast.

Almond Biscotti and English Breakfast Tea
Chai Pumpkin Seed Muffins and Oolong Tea
Orange Nut Whole Tea Scone with
Devonshire Cream and Black Tea
Cherry Almond Croissants and a Pot of Jasmine Tea
Strawberry Banana Tea Muffins and Chai

Almond Biscotti and English Breakfast Tea

❖ ❖ ❖

Making this Italian cookie is checked off my list of phobias. I prepared for my fear of baking biscotti, the double-baked cookie. I collected items including almonds, anise (a licorice extract used to flavor cookies), dark chocolate, and parchment paper. I was ready to make it happen even though I was entering unchartered waters.

3 cups all-purpose flour
3 teaspoons baking powder
½ cup European-style butter (you can use ¼ cup fruity olive oil)
1 cup white sugar, granulated
3 large organic eggs
1 teaspoon raw honey
1 teaspoon fresh orange juice
1 teaspoon anise extract
1 teaspoon vanilla extract
1½ cups chopped almonds

In a mixing bowl, combine flour and baking powder. Set aside. Cream butter and sugar in an electric mixer bowl at high speed until mixed well. Add eggs. Mix in dry ingredients (flour and baking powder). Add honey, juice, extracts, and almonds. Put flour on your hands, shape dough into two logs 8 to 12 inches long, 2½ inches wide and ½ to 1½ inches thick. On a parchment-covered cookie sheet place rolls. Bake at 350 degrees for about 25 minutes. Remove from oven and cool for about 10 minutes for a less crumbly cut. Slice rolls into ½-inch strips. Place cut side up on fresh parchment-papered cookie sheet. Put back into a 400-degree oven and bake till golden brown. Cool. Makes approximately 30 cookies (the amount varies depending on how big or small you slice the logs).

ICING

Mix ½ cup dark chocolate chips with ¼ cup half-and-half. Melt in microwave. Add ½ to 1 cup confectioners' sugar. Dip side of cookies into chocolate. Roll in almonds. Place in fridge till icing hardens. Store in container. Freezes well.

Chai Pumpkin Seed Muffins and Oolong Tea

❖ ❖ ❖

This creative recipe is a long-time favorite of mine given a new twist by adding chai and pumpkin seeds. Fresh out of the oven complemented with a cup of hot or iced oolong tea, it will make your day in the autumn.

1 cup each whole wheat flour and all-purpose flour
½ cup organic brown sugar
¼ cup white sugar
3 teaspoons baking powder
A dash of sea salt
2 teaspoons pumpkin pie spice
1 teaspoon chai, loose leaf (finely ground)
1 stick European-style butter, melted
½ cup canned pumpkin puree
½ cup organic half-and-half
2 eggs, brown
¾ cup shelled pumpkin seeds, chopped (save ¼ cup for sprinkling muffin tops)
Raw or confectioners' sugar for dusting muffin tops

In a bowl, combine flour, sugars, baking powder, salt, pumpkin pie spice, and chai. Set aside. In another bowl, mix butter, pumpkin, half-and-half, eggs, and seeds. Combine all ingredients and stir till well mixed. Use a ⅓-cup ice cream scoop to put batter into cupcake tins. Bake at 350 F for about 20 minutes or till golden brown and firm. Top with seeds and sugar. Makes 12. Serve warm with honey, organic jam, or cream cheese.

Orange Nut Whole Tea Scone
with Devonshire Cream and Black Tea

These scones were created by me and gleaned from a wide collection of my scone recipes. I adore this formula because the scones are soft, citrusy, and healthful with Greek yogurt, tea, dried fruit, and nuts. I like making the big circle scone instead of drop scones because it's easier and still rustic when cutting into wedges after it's baked.

2 cups cake flour
1 tablespoon baking powder
¼ cup granulated sugar
5 tablespoons European-style butter (cold cubes)
1 organic egg
⅔ cup half-and-half
1 teaspoon honey vanilla Greek yogurt
2 teaspoons brewed orange pekoe tea
1 teaspoon vanilla extract
2 tablespoons fresh orange rind, grated
¾–1 cup dried berries (blueberries or cranberries), chopped
½ cup hazelnuts, chopped
Raw sugar

Preheat oven to 350 degrees. In a bowl, mix flour, baking powder, and sugar. Add chunks of butter. In another bowl, combine egg, half-and-half, yogurt, tea, and vanilla and stir till mixed. Fold in rind, berries, and nuts. Put into lightly greased round baking dish (I used my favorite tart dish or you can use a round scone pan). Bake till golden brown, about 30 minutes. Sprinkle with sugar. Cool. Cut in triangle shapes like a pizza. Makes approximately 12. Serve with honey or cream cheese. (For a special touch, make an orange glaze. Mix confectioners' sugar with a bit of fresh orange juice and orange rind. Drizzle on tops of scones.) Serve with black tea.

DEVONSHIRE CREAM

For spreading on hearty scones or muffins, Devonshire cream is a fine sweet addition that you'll find served in tearooms. You can enjoy it in the comfort of your home with a cup of hot tea and edibles that call for a bit of creamy decadence.

⅛ cup sour cream
½ cup premium cream cheese
¼ cup confectioners' sugar
⅛ teaspoon pure vanilla extract

In a bowl combine sour cream, cream cheese, sugar, and vanilla. Whip until creamy. Serve immediately or refrigerate until use. Top with organic fruit jam for best flavor.

As a scone buff I can honestly tell you these light scones were enjoyed from the first to last bite—and after baking a batch the kitchen smelled like cotton candy. The layers of flavor—sweet, juicy strawberries, soft nuts, the tang of orange, and rich buttery taste—were a fine treat for the first day of spring. Two cups of green tea (I prefer chamomile or black but I'm expanding my tea collection) gave me the jump start to begin the new day, the new season. And I was smitten by starting out the morning with a scone, tea, and the new sound of chirping from a sole bird on the first day of spring.

Cherry Almond Croissants and Pot of Jasmine Tea

Croissants are a French pastry that has been made for centuries. But semi-homemade fruit and nut croissants, like these, are easy to make and taste sublime. The recipe below is one I tried and was surprised at the fresh and flaky homemade taste that pairs with a perfect pot of specialty tea.

Parchment paper
1 tube refrigerated croissant rolls, whole wheat [no trans fats]

8 tablespoons organic cherry jam
8 tablespoons fresh cherries, pitted, chopped
8 tablespoons almonds, sliced
Raw sugar
Cherries, fresh and whole (for garnish)
Cream cheese or clotted cream

Put a piece of parchment paper on a cookie sheet. Pop open package of rolls. On a flat surface unroll the eight precut triangle-shaped dough pieces. Put a tablespoon each of jam, cherries, and nuts on each triangle (the wide end). Roll into croissant shape. Sprinkle with almonds and sugar. Bake at 350 degrees for about 10 minutes or until golden brown. Cool. Serves eight. Pair with a pat of European-style butter or cream cheese, and fresh cherries to make these croissants even more decadent and eye-catching. Serve with jasmine tea.

Strawberry Banana Tea Muffins and Chai

Muffins paired with tea are a combination that is familiar. This is my own recipe, a spin-off of banana muffins I'd purchase after swimming at the resort pool. Homemade muffins, though, are just as good if not better at home with a freshly brewed cup of tea.

¼ cup oat bran
1 cup flour
¾ cup whole wheat pastry flour
1¼ teaspoon baking powder
¾ teaspoon baking soda
½ teaspoon salt
½ cup sugar
1 egg
⅓ cup Sciabica orange olive oil
½ teaspoon Danish pastry extract (Watkins)
1 cup banana, ripe, mashed (2 to 3 bananas)
½ cup raspberry or strawberry jam

In mixing bowl add bran, flours, baking powder, baking soda, salt, and sugar. Add egg, olive oil, extract, and banana. Stir just until mixed well. Turn into greased muffin pans, drop a teaspoon of jam on top of each muffin. Bake in a 375-degree oven for 15 to 20 minutes or until cake tester comes out clean from center. Makes 12. Serve with a cup of chai.

(*Courtesy: Baking Sensational Sweets with California Olive Oil* by Gemma Sanita Sciabica)

Tea-Infused Salads and Assorted Appetizers

Light salads and dinner salads with tea-infused dressings and/or appetizers are easy on the eyes and a cup of tea is bliss. When at home or traveling it is this type of treat that I love. Not only is it light but it's comforting, especially if served at afternoon tea or high tea. Either way it works like a continental breakfast.

Mediterranean Salad with Citrus Tea Vinaigrette
Mini Bruschettas and Fruit Tea
Organic Baby Spinach with Organic Tea Seed Oil Dressing
Stuffed Eggs and Green Tea
Vegetable Quiche and Darjeeling or Sencha

Mediterranean Salad with Citrus Tea Vinaigrette

Salads, like this one, are easy to make. This recipe, complete with the tea-infused vinaigrette, is mine and one I use whenever I want to drop a few pounds or detox my body after indulging in holiday foods.

½ cup mushrooms, chopped
½ cup tomatoes, diced
¼ cup green bell pepper, chopped
2 cups fresh greens (spring mix, baby spinach)
¼ cup roasted sunflower seeds, shelled
2 eggs, hard boiled, sliced
½ cup blue cheese, crumbled
Black pepper to taste

In a large bowl, toss mushrooms, tomatoes, and bell pepper. Fold in lettuce. Top with seeds, eggs, and cheese. Sprinkle with pepper. Makes

3–4 servings or 2 servings if main dish. It is perfect with a pot of green or white tea. (Use dressing below.)

CITRUS TEA VINAIGRETTE

4 citrus tea bags
½ cup boiling water
1 teaspoon honey
1 tablespoon red wine vinegar
⅛ cup fresh lemon juice
Salt to taste
1 tablespoon extra virgin olive oil

Place tea bags into a cup; pour in boiling water and let steep 10 minutes. Squeeze liquid out of tea bags and toss bags. Refrigerate for an hour. Combine cold tea and honey. Add the vinegar, lemon juice, and salt. Whisk oil into the ingredients. Drizzle on salad.

Mini Bruschettas and Fruit Tea

I have served this antipasto from Italy complete with fresh baguettes and olive oil as the perfect appetizer. Paired with a pitcher of iced tea or pot of hot tea, a high-quality fruit blend is sure to make this European snack a crowd pleaser.

Parchment paper
6–8 small slices baguette, sliced diagonally (¾ inch thick)
2 tablespoons European-style butter
1 tablespoon extra virgin olive oil
3 medium Roma tomatoes, seeded and chopped
2 tablespoons red onion, chopped
⅔ cup cheddar and Romano cheese, shredded
1 tablespoon each fresh mint and basil

Place bread slices on baking sheets (lined with parchment paper for easy cleanup). Spread bread lightly with butter and oil. Bake at 375 degrees for several minutes on each side till toasted. In a small bowl, combine tomatoes and onions. Spread even portions over toasted bread. Top with cheese. Bake for several minutes till cheese melts and bubbles. Garnish with mint and basil. Serves 3–4. Pair with fruit tea for the summer. (See "Healing Herbal Teas" chapter for tea beverage recipes.) In the fall, this recipe works well teamed up with a pot of hot black or green tea.

Organic Baby Spinach Salad with Organic Tea Seed Oil Dressing

❖ ❖ ❖

1 cup white wine vinegar
1 heaping tablespoon TCTC Glenburn Autumn Crescendo tea leaves
    (or an autumn harvest Darjeeling tea)
1 tablespoon honey
1 tablespoon chopped shallots
2 tablespoons cloves
2 tablespoons chopped garlic
1 tablespoon chopped fresh herbs such as a blend of thyme, sage, and
    tarragon
1 cup organic tea seed oil
Salt and fresh ground pepper to taste
1 small package fresh organic baby spinach
1 each of a variety of pears or apples, sliced thin
Feta cheese to taste

Bring the white wine vinegar to a boil. Remove from heat and add the tea leaves. Let sit until cool, then strain. Whisk together the infused vinegar, honey, shallots, cloves, garlic, and herbs, organic tea seed oil, salt, and pepper. Chill, before serving. Place the organic baby spinach in a bowl. Place the variety of fruit in a circular design over the spinach. Sprinkle with cheese. Makes 2 cups dressing, serving size 1 tablespoon.

(*Courtesy:* The Cozy Tea Cart)

Stuffed Eggs and Green Tea

❖ ❖ ❖

A pot of hot or cold tea, depending upon the season, was one of the beverages for the grown-ups when these eggs were served by my mother back when I was a toddler. Black tea, a staple in China, with lemon slices pairs well with eggs, ham, or crabmeat—all foods to eat in moderation and listed in the Oldways Mediterranean Diet Pyramid.

6 eggs, hard cooked
2 tablespoons sweet pickled relish
4 tablespoons ham, minced (or crabmeat)
1 tablespoon apple cider vinegar
1 tablespoon honey
1 tablespoon prepared mustard
¼ teaspoon Tabasco sauce
Salt and pepper to taste
Paprika to taste
6 pimento-stuffed olives for tops
2 tablespoons Marsala olive oil

Slice peeled, cooked eggs in half lengthwise, then carefully scoop yolks into a bowl. Place whites on a serving platter. In a bowl mix relish, meat, vinegar, honey, mustard, Tabasco sauce, spices, olives, and olive oil with yolks, then mash until blended. Using a spoon, fill each white with filling, rounding top, or use a pastry bag with ½-inch star tip. Pipe filling into whites, and sprinkle stuffed eggs with paprika; place an olive slice on center of each. Serves 12 halves. Serve with English Afternoon tea.

(*Courtesy: Cooking with California Olive Oil: Recipes from the Heart for the Heart* by Gemma Sanita Sciabica)

Vegetable Quiche with Darjeeling or Sencha
❖ ❖ ❖

Quiche, a rich but good-for-you custard pie infused with cheese and vegetables, offers choices: eat it any time of day, hot or cold. It may have French roots but it's also a favorite here in America. I give this recipe of mine a Mediterranean spin. My mother would be proud. And yes, I've finally acquired a taste for fresh spinach. So, turn up the heat or stoke the fire and cuddle up. Enjoy! And yes, I know for a fact real men eat quiche!

1 tablespoon olive oil
1 tablespoon European-style butter
2 tablespoons garlic olive oil
¼ cup red onion, diced
1¼ cup organic fresh baby spinach, thinly sliced
1¼ cups mix of green and red bell pepper, zucchini, chopped
1 teaspoon herbs (a blend of fresh basil, rosemary, sage, thyme, and
   lavender)
4 organic brown eggs, beaten
1 cup organic half-and-half
1 teaspoon extra virgin olive oil
1 (9-inch) store-bought refrigerated pie crust (or mini tart shells)
1 cup low-fat mozzarella, shredded
2 slices mozzarella, chopped
12 cherry tomatoes, sliced in half

In a skillet, melt garlic olive oil and butter. Stir-fry onion, spinach, bell pepper, add herbs. Set aside. In a mixing bowl, beat eggs, add half-and-half. Brush olive oil on uncooked pie crust. Top with half of veggie mixture. Sprinkle with half of cheese. Repeat. Pour milk-egg mixture on top. Place tomato halves on top. Bake at 400 degrees for about 45 minutes or till golden brown and firm. Makes 8–10 servings. Pairs well with Darjeeling or Sencha teas. (Mini tart shells can be found at your supermarket. Follow directions for the crusts and bake filling for approximately 25 minutes or until firm.)

Assorted Finger Tea Sandwiches

Ah, tea sandwiches. These mini delights are popular during afternoon tea more than high tea. The way to enjoy healthy finger tea sandwiches is to use fresh ingredients, including herbs and spices, like you'll find in the Mediterranean diet. This is the time to think outside of the breadbox and use different breads—whole grain, baguettes, raisin-nut, Hawaiian sweet rolls—to make it fun and different. Using biscuit or cookie cutters to create a variety of shapes including circles and flowers is pleasing to the eye.

Cold Tuna, Cracked Wheat Bread
Cucumber and Watercress Tea Sandwiches
Goat Cheese/Baby Spinach on Brioche
Grilled Cheese and Tomato Triangle Sandwich
Organic Egg Salad on Croissants
Peanut Butter and Honey Flowers

Cold Tuna, Cracked Wheat Bread

Tuna sandwiches are a popular, flavorful favorite and easy to make. This recipe of mine has a refined European twist (with olive oil, fresh basil, and red wine vinegar) to make it a super find on any tiered plate of finger sandwiches.

1 6-ounce can albacore tuna, drained and flaked
2 tablespoons olive oil mayonnaise dressing
¼ cup red onion, chopped
2–4 fresh basil leaves
¼ cup lettuce, chopped
4 slices cracked wheat bread, cold
¼ cup Roma tomatoes, chopped

1 teaspoon red wine vinegar
Pepper and sea salt to taste

In a small bowl combine tuna and mayonnaise, mix well. Add onion and basil. Place lettuce on bread slice, then place some of the tuna mixture on top of the lettuce, and top with tomatoes. Drizzle with vinegar. Top with bread slice. Repeat. Cut off crusts. Use a cookie cutter (round, flower-shaped) and place on plate. *Note: Put bread in freezer to make it easier to cut pretty shapes. Serves 2.

Cucumber and Watercress Tea Sandwiches

When I made these dainty sandwiches, I wasn't sure if they would be my cup of tea. Surprisingly, they were tasty with the fresh bread, chives, and real butter. Perhaps it's not a sandwich well received in a man cave, but it can do well in a she-cave.

4 slices light rye bread (put in freezer so easier to cut in neat shapes)
2 tablespoons sea salt butter, melted
4 tablespoons whipped cream cheese
½ Roma tomato, sliced
1 tablespoon fresh chives, rough chop
½ large cucumber, remove skin (drain on paper towel, blot water)

Remove crusts of chilled bread (use sharp knife). Spread with butter, cream cheese, and top with tomato slices. Sprinkle chives on top. Place cucumber slices. Top with bread slices. Cut in rectangle or triangle shapes or use cookie cutters for different forms. Refrigerate. Serves 4.

Goat Cheese/Baby Spinach on Brioche

4 slices brioche (a rich French bread with egg and butter)
1 cup goat cheese, soft
1 cup baby spinach, chopped
¼ cup black olives, seeded, sliced
¼ cup sun-dried tomatoes
Sea salt and fresh ground pepper to taste

On a plate place 2 slices bread. Spread cheese, top with spinach, olives, and tomatoes. Sprinkle with salt and pepper. Place 2 slices of bread on top. Cut in 4 squares per sandwich. Serves 2–4.

Grilled Cheese and Tomato Triangle Sandwich

2–3 tablespoons European-style butter, cubed
4 slices whole wheat sourdough bread
4 slices cheddar cheese, sliced
¾ cup Italian cheeses (your choice), shredded
1 large Roma tomato, sliced

Heat a large frying pan over medium heat. Melt butter. Place slices of bread on one side in pan. Top with cheese. Once cheese melts, place remaining slices of bread on top of each sandwich. Press sandwiches with spatula. Toast sandwiches on both sides to melt cheese. Add tomatoes. Remove when golden brown and crispy. Cut off crusts. Cut in 4 triangles per each sandwich. Serves 2.

Organic Egg Salad on Croissants

4 large organic eggs, hard-boiled
¼ cup olive oil mayonnaise dressing
¼ cup celery, chopped
2 tablespoons chives
1 tablespoon red onion, chopped
4 small whole wheat croissants
½ teaspoon ground pepper
Sea salt to taste
½ cup organic spring lettuce

In a bowl, mix eggs with mayonnaise, celery, chives, and onion. Put in refrigerator for at least 30 minutes. Place lettuce on sliced fresh croissants (store bought or from a bakery is easier). Top with egg salad, sprinkle pepper and salt. Top with other bread slice. Serves 2–4.

Peanut Butter and Honey Flowers

4 slices raisin or date nut bread
2 tablespoons premium peanut butter
2 teaspoons clover honey

Place bread slices on a plate. Spread soft peanut butter on 2 slices. Top with honey. Put on top of second slice of bread. (Use chilled slices.) Cut crusts. Use flower-shaped cookie cutters. Serves 2–4.

Savory Dishes

Tea-infused entrees are nothing new but they may be new to you. Tea leaves, brewed, ground, or used whole, can enhance a dish, whether it is lean meat, vegetables, fish, or poultry. There are delicious recipes in this section, from the Pork Tenderloin with Tea to Scallops in Black Tea Marinade, that'll wow your taste buds as you step out of your comfort zone and enjoy something flavorful with an exotic flair.

Crab Cakes with a Pot of White Tea
Earl Grey Waffles with Oven Fried Chicken
Pork Tenderloin with Tea
Orange Squeeze Tea Spiced Carrots
Scallops in Black Tea Marinade
Tea-Infused Mushroom Soup

Crab Cakes with a Pot of White Tea

½ pound crab meat, fresh
2 tablespoons fine corn meal
½ cup bread crumbs (Japanese bread crumbs, panko)
Sea salt and white pepper to taste
2 eggs
¼ cup celery, chopped
½ cup shallots or green onions, chopped
2 tablespoons lemon juice
2 garlic cloves, minced
¼ cup pimientos, minced
⅓ cup Sciabica's or Marsala Extra Virgin Olive Oil (save a bit for drizzling)
1 tablespoon jalapeño, minced
Dash of Worcestershire sauce
Lemon wedges for garnish

Combine crab meat, corn meal, bread crumbs, salt and pepper, eggs, celery, shallots or green onions, lemon juice, garlic cloves, pimientos, olive oil, jalapeño, and Worcestershire sauce in mixing bowl. Shape mixture into patties. Place in refrigerator for 20 minutes. Lightly grease baking pan, add olive oil, place patties on bottom. Drizzle with a little olive oil on top of cakes. Bake in a 350-degree oven for 20 to 30 minutes or until golden. Serve with lemon wedges and avocado salsa if desired. Serves 4.

Author's Note: You can drizzle a tea sauce on top; mix 1 tablespoon of ½ cup brewed chamomile tea and 1 tablespoon fresh lemon juice.

(*Courtesy: Cooking with California Olive Oil: Recipes from the Heart for the Heart* by Gemma Sanita Sciabica)

Earl Grey Waffles with Oven Fried Chicken

4 tablespoons European-style butter (put aside an extra bit for cooked waffles)
2 organic brown eggs
1 cup low-fat buttermilk
3 Earl Grey tea bags
1 cup all-purpose flour or whole wheat flour
¾ teaspoon baking powder
2 tablespoons granulated sugar (or 1 tablespoon honey)
A pinch of cinnamon and nutmeg
Maple syrup for topping
½ cup fresh berries

Use a nonstick waffle iron (no oil or butter needed). In a mixing bowl, combine melted butter and eggs. Set aside. In a saucepan heat buttermilk with tea bags until hot but not boiling. Remove tea bags, cool. Add butter, eggs, flour, baking powder, sugar, honey, cinnamon, and nutmeg. Pour half batter on heated waffle grid. Close lid and bake till steam rises. Place waffle on plate and repeat. Serves two (double recipes for four). Top with syrup and chicken (see below).

Oven Fried Chicken

2 pounds chicken pieces, boneless, skinless
1 egg slightly beaten
½ cup bread crumbs
Salt, pepper to taste
½ cup corn meal or farina
Cayenne to taste
½ cup basil and/or parsley
⅓ cup nuts of your choice, ground
⅓ cup Romano cheese, grated
4 garlic cloves, minced
½ cup Marsala olive oil

Pound chicken pieces to about ½ inch thick. In pie plate add egg. In another plate mix bread crumbs, salt, pepper, corn meal, cayenne, basil, parsley, nuts, cheese, and garlic. Dip each chicken piece in egg on both sides, then in crumb mixture on each side. Lightly grease baking sheet, drizzle with a little olive oil. Lay chicken pieces in single layer or slightly overlapping in pan, then drizzle with olive oil. Bake in 350-degree oven, covered with foil for 15 minutes. Turn chicken on second side, bake another 15 to 20 minutes or until golden brown and tender. Use instant read thermometer. Serves 4 to 6. (Author's Suggestion: Serve with Sweet Tea or Iced Tea—Recipes are in this book in previous chapters.)

(*Courtesy:* Gemma Sanita Sciabica, *Cooking with California Olive Oil: Popular Recipes*)

Pork Tenderloin with Tea

This recipe was created for me by my dear friend Gemma. My mother used to make tender and juicy pork chops with a side dish of scalloped potatoes for Sunday dinners. While I'm a vegetarian, I couldn't pass on sharing this tea-infused meat creation. And the Oldways Mediterranean Diet does include pork (in moderation).

¾ cup cereal (rice or corn flakes, crushed)
¼ cup grated Romano cheese
¼ teaspoon cardamom
1 tablespoon dried tea powder (your choice of a spiced tea)
3–3½ pounds pork tenderloin
1 egg white, lightly beaten
⅓ cup olive oil
Grated peel of 1 lemon

Preheat oven to 350 degrees. In shallow bowl combine cereal, cheese, cardamom, and dried tea powder. Roll pork in egg white, all around, then in cereal mixture. Drizzle with olive oil and grated peel of 1 lemon. Place in lightly greased roasting pan. Bake until instant-read thermometer for meat reaches about 160 degrees. Serve with stewed prunes, apples, or fruit of your choice.

(*Courtesy*: Gemma Sanita Sciabica)

Orange Squeeze Tea Spiced Carrots

I've always liked raw carrots, but a cooked carrot recipe is something I'm not used to cooking. This recipe comes from a seasoned tea master and tea just may be the ingredient that convinces me to make an exception and add it to my cooked vegetable favorite dishes.

2 cups water
2 tablespoons sweet orange black tea (TCTC Orange Squeeze Tea)
4 cups carrots, chopped
1 stick butter
Rind of 1 orange
1 teaspoon fresh ginger
1 teaspoon coriander
2 tablespoons Grand Marnier

Boil the water in a medium covered pot, along with the orange black tea. Steep for 5 minutes. Sift the tea from the water. Place the carrots in the tea-infused water and steam until tender. Drain carrots and set aside. Combine the butter, orange rind, ginger, coriander, and Grand Marnier, and cook over low heat until the butter melts. Add the carrots. Serves 4–5.

(*Courtesy*: The Cozy Tea Cart.)

Scallops in Black Tea Marinade

This fish recipe is easy to follow and has an earthy, California coastal vibe to it. It needs a loaf of French bread or baguette slices dipped in olive oil or spread with real butter, and it's a Hemingway-type noteworthy feast I'd be proud to serve to family, friends, and solo for a special occasion. (I used white tea.)

3 tablespoons blend of Breakfast tea, a blend of Sri Lankan, Kenyan and Assam (TCTC Bengal Breakfast Tea)
2 cups of boiled water
1 medium onion, finely chopped
Salt and pepper
1–1½ pounds scallops

Marinating time is overnight. Brew the tea in the boiled water. Let steep for 20 minutes. Strain the leaves and let the liquid cool to room temperature. Combine the finely chopped onion with salt and pepper to taste. Add the scallops to the onion mixture. Pour the tea over the scallops and marinate overnight in the fridge. Before serving, drain the marinade. Thread the scallops on skewers and cook over a pre-heated grill for 3–4 minutes on each side until cooked through. Serve over a combination of spinach and arugula and drizzle with organic lemon juice or leave on the skewer and serve as an appetizer. Serves 4.

(*Courtesy*: The Cozy Tea Cart)

Tea-Infused Mushroom Soup

1 tablespoon organic green tea leaves (Guo Lu green tea leaves or
   rolled green tea)
6 cups water
1 cup dried porcini mushrooms
3 cups boiling water
2 tablespoons organic tea seed oil
1 large onion, chopped
3 cloves garlic, chopped
2 stocks celery, finely chopped
3 large carrots, diced
15 ounces fresh tomatoes, diced
½ cup fresh crimini mushrooms, sliced
½ cup fresh shitake mushrooms, sliced
1 tablespoon soy sauce
1 tablespoon chopped rosemary
1 tablespoon chopped fresh sage
Diced scallions for garnish

Steep the green tea in six cups 160 degrees water for 5 minutes. Do
not strain. Set aside. Steep the dried mushrooms in 3 cups of boiling
water for 20 minutes. Strain the mushrooms but save the liquid to add
to the soup. Slice the mushrooms. In a large pot, heat the organic tea
seed oil, onion, garlic, celery, carrots, and tomatoes over medium heat
until soft, about 10 minutes. Add the steeped green tea and leaves to
the pot. Add the steeped dried mushrooms, then reserved mushroom
liquid, soy sauce, rosemary, and sage to the pot. Simmer for 2 hours.
Serve with a sprinkle of the diced scallions. Serves 4–5.

(*Courtesy*: The Cozy Tea Cart)

Signature Tea Desserts

Apple Chamomile Tea Cake
Earl Grey Baked Rice Pudding
Gingerbread Tea Cupcakes with Matcha Frosting
Harvest Pumpkin Spice Tea Bundt Cake
Royal Chocolate Chai Mousse
Vanilla Black Tea–Infused Lemon Pound Cake Squares

Apple Chamomile Tea Cake

Apple cake recipes with fresh apples, an autumn favorite, go back centuries. This recipe, my own, has served me throughout the years but I continue to make minor tweaks, and this time around it's infused with a bit of a special chamomile tea blend.

2½ cups cake flour
¼ cup granulated white sugar
½ cup light brown sugar
2 teaspoons baking soda
1 teaspoon cinnamon
½ teaspoon allspice
½ teaspoon nutmeg
1 tablespoon apple cinnamon chamomile, finely ground loose leaf
 (The Cozy Tea Cart)
1 stick European sea salt butter (save 1 tablespoon to grease
 cake dish)
½ cup Granny Smith apples, cored, chopped, unpeeled
½ cup raisins
2 eggs
2 tablespoons honey (optional)
Sea salt caramel gelato

In a large bowl, mix the flour, sugars, baking soda, spices, and tea. Add cold butter chunks, apples, raisins, eggs, and honey. Stir until mixed. Spoon batter into a buttered 8 x 8-inch baking dish or pan. Bake at 325 degrees for 45 minutes or until firm and light golden. Cool. Sprinkle with confectioners' sugar. Cut into squares. Top with a small mini scoop of sea salt caramel gelato. Serves 16.

Earl Grey Baked Rice Pudding

❖ ❖ ❖

This dessert is a gem for brown rice fans. Rice pudding is a popular dish around the globe. Created from rice combined with milk and other stuff like raisins and cinnamon, it can be sweet cold or hot. Since the temperatures are still cool in the Sierra, I baked this dish and it brought back bittersweet memories of budget-friendly comfort food.

1¼ cups cooked brown rice
2 eggs (organic brown), beaten
2½ cups organic half-and-half
½ cup organic low-fat milk
¼ cup granulated sugar
2 teaspoons honey
1 teaspoon vanilla extract
1 cup golden raisins
1 tablespoon cinnamon
1 tablespoon Earl Grey leaves, finely ground (Harney & Sons)
1 teaspoon nutmeg
European-style butter (to grease baking dish)
Lemon and orange slices, cinnamon sticks, mint for garnish
    (optional)

In a bowl, combine rice, eggs, half-and-half, milk, sugar, honey, vanilla, raisins, cinnamon, and tea. Lightly grease with butter an 8 x 8 baking dish (or use ramekins). Bake at 325 degrees in a pan of water (about 2 or 3 inches) for 1½ hours until golden brown. Top immediately with nutmeg. Serve warm. Garnish as you wish. Makes approximately 6–8 servings. Serve with a pot of jasmine tea in the autumn or winter.

Gingerbread Tea Cupcakes
with Matcha Frosting

❖ ❖ ❖

One New Year's Eve, I cooked black-eyed peas for my elderly neighbor, per her request. She believed the coin-shaped legumes could bring good fortune for the upcoming year. The Deep South tradition made the silver-haired woman giggle and smile like a young girl. For old time's sake, I'll make New Year's vows each year and make cupcakes, like these (the round shape of the cakes and fruit), which may bring luck.

CAKES

¾ cup dark brown sugar
¾ cup molasses
½ cup European-style butter (1 stick), melted (save a tablespoon for greasing baking dish)
2 organic brown eggs
2½ cups all-purpose flour
2 teaspoons baking soda
1 tablespoon ground ginger
1 teaspoon cinnamon
½ teaspoon allspice
1 cup hot water
½ cup crystallized ginger pieces
¾ to 1 cup pomegranate seeds (1 pomegranate)
2 teaspoons orange rind (optional)

In a large mixing bowl, combine sugar, molasses, butter, and eggs. Stir until smooth. Set aside. In a medium-sized bowl, mix flour, baking soda, ginger, cinnamon, and allspice. Combine sugar, molasses, butter, and egg mixture to dry ingredients. Add water. Mix thoroughly. Fold in ginger pieces. Set aside. Slice pomegranate in four pieces and place in water for five minutes. Pick out seeds, drain. Add pomegranate seeds and mix lightly.

Use a mini-cupcake pan (grease with oil or butter or nonstick baking spray). Pour batter into each hole (use small ice cream scoop or tablespoon to make the mini-cupcakes uniform in size so they will bake evenly). Bake at 350 degrees for about 15–20 minutes or until the tops are firm. Do not overbake. Cool. Makes approximately 20 mini-cupcakes.

MATCHA FROSTING

1 cup confectioners' sugar
3 tablespoons organic 2% low-fat milk
¼–½ teaspoon organic premium matcha tea powder (Full Leaf Tea Company)
½ teaspoon pure vanilla extract

In a small mixing bowl, combine sugar, milk, tea powder, and vanilla. Stir well or blend with a mixer until smooth and creamy. Frost gingerbread squares piped with creamy green tea frosting. Serve cupcakes with a side of fresh sliced peaches.

Harvest Pumpkin Spice Tea Bundt Cake

Welcome to autumn. It's the ideal time to splurge on a slice of warm pumpkin spice tea cake and mug of hot tea. Meet Mr. Bundt cake. It's a must-have fall dessert baked in a Bundt pan—a round shape with grooves and a hole in the middle. A Bundt pan comes from Europe but it's been popular for decades in the United States, too. Not only is it versatile (as a big or small tea cake), to me there is nothing so delicious as a bit of warm, spicy pumpkin cake during the Harvest Moon and Mother Nature's serene seasonal changes.

This semi-homemade cake is moist, thanks to the flavorful pumpkin of my favorite season. The earthy spices give the Bundt cake a fall-like jump start with its spicy scent in the kitchen; and the chocolate adds a rich, creamy texture and bittersweet taste. Not to forget the smooth cream cheese icing with a nice crunch from raw sugar. If you're looking for a harvest cake your quest is over. This cake will win you over with its unique beauty and timely nature.

1–2 tablespoons butter (for greasing pan or mini-Bundt cakes pan)
2 extra-large organic brown eggs
6 tablespoons butter or olive oil (I used unsalted European-style)
1 spice cake mix (premium brand without trans fats)
2 tablespoons all-purpose flour (optional: use this if you live in high
    altitude)
1 cup water
1 cup canned pumpkin puree
1 teaspoon pumpkin spice
1 teaspoon ground cinnamon spice tea (Harney & Sons Hot
    Cinnamon Spice Loose Tea)
½ teaspoon spice tea, finely ground (Bigelow)
½–¾ cup dark chocolate chips
Raw sugar to taste

Butter Bundt pan (or use a mini-Bundt cakes pan for tea cakes) and set aside. In a mixing bowl, beat eggs and melted European-style butter. Stir in cake mix and flour. Add water and pumpkin. Sprinkle in pumpkin spice and spice teas and stir. Fold in chocolate. Mix until batter is smooth without lumps. Using a large spatula, put batter into pan, smooth so it's flat. Bake at 350 degrees for 40 minutes or till a knife inserted in the middle of the cake comes out clean and is firm to touch. Cool for 10 minutes, then place a plate on top and turn over. Cool and drizzle frosting on top of slightly warm cake. Sprinkle with raw sugar. Serves 12–14. Serve with a pot of black or green and white tea with cinnamon sticks as a garnish.

CREAM CHEESE FROSTING

1½–2 cups whipped cream cheese
2 tablespoons European-style butter
1½ cups confectioners' sugar
¼ cup organic 2% low-fat milk
1 capful vanilla extract
1 teaspoon lemon rind
Walnuts, chopped (garnish)

Mix cream cheese and butter. Stir in sugar. Add milk and vanilla. Blend in mixer until creamy. Fold in rind. Drizzle frosting over the top of the cooled cake and let it drip down the sides. Sprinkle top with nuts.

Royal Chai Chocolate Mousse

Chocolate mousse, a decadent dessert, is a must-have on my tea menu any day of the year. I chose the egg-less no-cook method. This rich chocolate mousse is a keeper year-round. The first bite is creamy and chocolaty. Chai adds an earthy, spicy flavor married with the fluffy whipped cream topping. Berries add a sweet freshness. If you want an easier recipe, use store-bought ready-made whipped cream (Cool Whip) for a thicker texture that'll please the less sophisticated palate.

1 cup premium all-natural milk chocolate chips, 31% cacao
   (Ghirardelli)
½ cup half-and-half
2 tablespoons European-style butter, melted
2 teaspoons chai, strong brew (Harney & Sons)
1½ cups heavy whipping cream (save ¼ cup for garnish)
1 capful pure vanilla extract
¼ cup confectioners' sugar
Extra whipped cream
Chocolate shavings (Ghirardelli dark chocolate bar, grated)
Mint, fresh sprigs

In a bowl pour one cup of chocolate chips. Place in microwave and melt. (Keep a close watch on it. Do not overcook. Stir until smooth.) Set aside. In another bowl, combine half-and-half and butter (microwave until butter is melted). Cool. Mix into chocolate. (At first it will look lumpy but stir and it will turn creamy and smooth.) Fold in chai. (Follow instructions on product.) Set aside. In a chilled mixing bowl pour whipping cream. Mix on high until it is a thick, creamy texture. (Warning: This can take a while. Use a cold bowl and beaters.) Add vanilla and sugar (it does need the sweet flavor). Fold ½ cup whipping cream into chocolate. Add the rest and stir until it's a creamy mousse. Pour into ramekins or small glasses. Place in refrigerator for 3 hours to firm. Top with whipped cream. Garnish with chocolate shavings, mint sprigs, and berries. *Note: A ready-made Cool Whip topping makes the texture fluffier if you don't have the time or desire to make whipped cream. Serves approximately 4. Pairs nicely with hot or iced jasmine or orange spice tea.

Vanilla Black Tea–Infused
Lemon Pound Cake Squares

❖ ❖ ❖

This is my recipe that is one to use when there isn't enough time in the day but you want to bake for that aroma in the kitchen, to be able to eat something fresh out of the oven, tea-infused, and paired with fruit and a cup of tea. The cake is buttery and moist so it doesn't need a rich glaze or frosting.

1 box premium lemon pound cake mix
¾ cup brewed tea (Harney & Sons vanilla black flavored loose leaf)
12 tablespoons butter, melted (save a teaspoon for greasing baking dish)
2 teaspoons lemon rind
¼ cup confectioners' sugar
Fresh strawberries, ¼ cup for each serving

Preheat oven to 350 degrees. In a bowl mix cake mix, tea, butter, and lemon rind. Pour into an 8 x 8 butter-greased baking dish. Bake for approximately 45–55 minutes or until firm. Remove and cool. Sprinkle with sugar. Top with berries. Makes about 20 small squares. Serve with black, white, or green tea.

Note: If you live in high altitude like I do, add 1 tablespoon all-purpose flour, and a few extra tablespoons of tea.

Assorted Candy and Cookies

Chai Petite Peanut Butter Cookies
Cinnamon Tea Chocolate Bark
Old Fashioned Molasses-Vanilla Tea Cookies
Orange Spice Tea–Infused Macaroons
Russian Tea Cookies

Chai Petite Peanut Butter Cookies

My mom baked large old-fashioned peanut butter cookies, the dark-colored kind because of the usage of dark brown sugar, and made a crisscross imprint (with a fork) on top. This is my adapted recipe, which creates a smaller, lighter colored cookie (using light brown sugar), European-style butter, autumn spices—and chai. These bite-size cookies boast an imperfect look—a rustic delight that gives a taste of home-made with present-day flavors that mesh with the 20th century.

2½ cups all-purpose flour
1½ teaspoon baking soda
1½ teaspoons (each) ground ginger and cinnamon
1 teaspoon chai, ground leaves (Harney & Sons)
⅓ cup European-style sea salt butter, soft
1 cup low-sodium, all-natural peanut butter, creamy
¼ cup white granulated sugar
½ cup light brown sugar
1 brown egg
1 teaspoon pure vanilla extract
Mediterranean Sea salt

Preheat oven to 400 degrees. In a bowl, combine flour, baking soda, ginger, cinnamon, and chai. Set aside. Add butter and peanut butter, white and brown sugars. Mix in egg and vanilla. Combine all ingredients and mix well. (It will be crumbly.) Form cookie dough into a snakelike roll and wrap in parchment paper. Chill for at least an hour. Slice dough into ¼-inch slices. Roll into petite balls and place on a cookie sheet lined with parchment paper. Use the bottom of a cup to flatten the balls. Place crisscross marks with fork on top of balls. Bake for about 8–10 minutes. Once out of the oven sprinkle half the cookies with Mediterranean Sea salt and the other half with jam. This way you'll have the best of both worlds. Makes about 3 dozen.

Cinnamon Tea Chocolate Bark

I've always loved this recipe, one I have used every fall and holiday season. It's easy and quick to make, pretty, and boasts a rustic look like peanut brittle.

8 ounces premium baking bar or chips, white chocolate
¼ teaspoon orange or lemon rind
½–1 teaspoon Hot Cinnamon Tea (Harney & Sons), ground loose leaves
½ cup hazelnuts or almonds, roughly chopped

Melt half chocolate (the bar makes a smoother bark than chips but both work) in a microwave for about 30 seconds, stir occasionally until semi-melted. (A double boiler is another way to melt the chocolate.) Add the rest of chocolate and stir until smooth and glossy. (Watch carefully so chocolate does not burn.) Stir in ground citrus rind and tea. Use a spice or coffee grinder for a rough or fine chop (both types work). Spread mixture onto a nonstick flat cookie sheet (or line pan with parchment paper so bark doesn't stick) and shape into a rectangle. Sprinkle with nuts. Chill in refrigerator for 30 minutes or until firm.

Take out and pick up entire candy slab, place on plate. Break into square pieces (it looks rustic instead of perfect squares). Package a few pieces in cellophane bags and tie with ribbon or put in a container and cover with a lid. Makes approximately 10–12 pieces. Store in the refrigerator (the flavorful pieces go fast). (Author's Note: To mix it up, try using milk or dark chocolate with Earl Grey and crushed peppermint candy or lavender tea leaves with white chocolate.)

Old Fashioned Molasses-Vanilla Tea Cookies

These classic cookies inspired by my childhood store-bought favorites found in the bear cookie jar on the kitchen countertop are pretty and chewy with the classic cracked look. The citrus zest and elegant vanilla frosting provides a fresh scent and taste paired with the warm spices. These molasses cookies paired with a hot cup of chamomile tea in autumn and fall or a lemony iced tea in spring and summer is perfect. Munching on a homemade cookie (or two) will provide me, and you, a sweet touch year-round.

½ cup European-style butter, unsalted, melted
¾ cup brown sugar
¼ cup granulated sugar
1 brown egg
¼ cup molasses
2½ cups all-purpose flour
2 teaspoons baking soda
1½ teaspoons ginger
1 teaspoon allspice
1 teaspoon pure vanilla extract
1 vanilla bean, scraped
2 tablespoons lemon zest
½ cup raw sugar

In a bowl, combine butter, sugars, egg, and molasses. Pour mixture into dry ingredients of flour, baking soda, ginger, and allspice. Add vanilla extract, vanilla bean, and lemon zest. Stir until the mix forms a dough. Place onto parchment paper and cover. Shape into a snakelike form and put into fridge for a couple of hours. Cut into ½-inch slices; shape into small- to medium-sized balls. Roll half the balls in ½ cup raw organic sugar. Leave the other half plain to frost. Place on cookie sheet lined with parchment paper. Bake at 375 degrees for about 10 minutes. Do not overbake. Makes 24 small-medium cookies.

VANILLA FROSTING

Combine 2 cups confectioners' sugar, about ¼ cup of 2% organic reduced fat milk, ½ teaspoon pure vanilla extract, and vanilla bean. Stir well. Frost tops of plain cookies and sprinkle with natural raw sugar.

Orange Spice Tea–Infused Macaroons

Any season these coconut macaroons bake nicely in the early morning when the air is cooler before a hot summer day or on a chilly autumn afternoon. Truly, these cookies are fail-proof to make whether you're a kid or adult. The moist texture, burst of citrus notes, and chewy cookie is good and the look is great. You'll be proud to show off these homemade cookies with a decadent chocolaty twist to your family and friends.

½ cup all-purpose flour (King Arthur flour)
⅛ teaspoon cream of tartar (optional)
¼ cup granulated white sugar
⅛ teaspoon sea salt
7 ounces sweetened condensed milk
1 capful each almond extract and pure vanilla extract
4½–5 cups sweetened coconut, premium
4 egg whites
1 teaspoon orange or lemon rind (optional)
½ cup premium dark chocolate chips or bar pieces (and/or white
    chocolate or milk chocolate)
Confectioners' sugar (for dusting) (optional)

In a large bowl, combine flour, cream of tartar, sugar, salt, milk, flavorings, and coconut. Set aside. In a mixing bowl beat egg whites until stiff. Fold in coconut mixture. Add rind. Use ⅓ cup ice cream scoop or 1 teaspoon (shaped like a cone or pyramid), and place cookie dough on ungreased cookie sheet or line with parchment paper. Bake at 325 degrees for 12–15 minutes (when the tops are light golden brown). Remove immediately. Cool and dip bottoms in melted chocolate and/

or dust some with confectioners' sugar. Makes about three dozen cookies, depending on your preferred size. Store in airtight container and put in fridge or freezer. These adorable cookies are best warm fresh out of the oven. (Caveat: Savor in moderation due to its sugar and saturated fat.)

Once I placed each cookie on the sheet I sensed this recipe was a keeper. I peeked in the oven after five minutes and the mounds did not spread. The first bite was cookie heaven: crispy on the outside, moist and chewy on the inside. These macaroons are ideal for February—the romantic Valentine's Day month, especially with dark chocolate on the bottom or swirled on top. I used my own measurements and fine ingredients and ignored umpteen recipes (some called for too much condensed milk, no flour or too much sugar or not enough coconut). This decadent cookie is for all seasons. Chocolate and tea pairings work well with teas—iced or hot. Try matcha, Earl Grey, or a citrusy herbal tea in a glaze for different seasons and you'll be pleased. These cookies freeze well. Glaze with tea-infused chocolate for a fresh taste once thawed.

Russian Tea Cookies

Inspired by the holidays when I was living in Eugene, Oregon, this popular dessert cookie with Russian roots goes back to the Middle Ages. It's a simple confection to create but it's big on flavor, and its pretty appearance and light but crunchy texture has a sweet sophistication, especially paired with a steaming cup of English Breakfast or green tea. During my past pre-winter days in Eugene, Oregon, on a snow day, I'd make a batch of Russian Tea Cookies and package boxes of the gems to relatives. These mini mound-shaped cookies require few ingredients and are sweet delights year-round paired with tea. I dedicate these cookies to my grandmother and her recipe that I treasure *and* how she taught me the art of paying it forward with tea and treats.

½ cup soft butter, European-style with sea salt
1 cup cake flour (an extra 2 tablespoons in high altitude), sifted
1 cup confections' sugar (reserve ½ cup for rolling cookies)

½ cup walnuts, fine or rough chop
1 capful of pure vanilla extract
1 teaspoon fresh lemon juice
Optional: ½ teaspoon ground tea leaves (lavender or Earl Grey)

In a mixing bowl, cream butter and flour, add sugar, and blend. Add nuts, vanilla, and lemon juice. Add tea. Chill 30 minutes. On a parchment-lined cookie sheet place 1 inch rolled cookies. Do not press. Bake at 325 for 18–20 minutes. Roll in sugar. Cool. Roll cookies in sugar once again. Store in airtight container. Serves 12–16.

Specialty Tea Menu Suggestions

BLACK TEA

French Vanilla Loose Leaf Black Tea

A Ceylon black tea blend with the classic European flavor of French vanilla

ORGANIC EARL GREY

Organic black tea leaves, essence of organic bergamot

GREEN TEA

Organic green tea leaves, organic jasmine flowers

HERBAL TEA

Chamomile Blend Tea

Chamomile flowers lend their superb calming virtues to this blend of delicate sweet notes of citrus and linden, catnip, and calendula

ROOBIOS TEA

Coconut Custard, Rooibos, coconut shred

WHITE TEA

Bai Mu Dan

Chinese white tea from the Fujian province; smooth, airy and lightly sweet flavor with hints of honey and vanilla

White Velvet

Whole leaf Mutan white tea from China infused with vanilla, a hint of rose flavor

TEA-CENTRIC HEALING HINTS TO STEEP

✓ There are an infinite number of standout tea companies in the United States and around the world; my close-up encounter with many different brands taught me well that there is more than tea bags—from loose leaf to sachets—and I learned the art of grinding leaves and brewing a pot of tea.

✓ Visiting everything from tea shops and tearooms to specialty stores, health food stores, and grocery stores to purchase fine tea is a worthwhile experience . . .

✓ . . . And discovering different types of teas from different regions can be done via the Internet with the click of your mouse.

✓ Keep in mind, tea companies come and go, merge and change players—but tea is here to stay, play a role in your recipes, and stand alone, and its demand will likely grow throughout the coming years.

Final Tea Notes

I say let the world go to hell, but I should always have my tea.
—Fyodor Dostoyevsky, *Notes from the Underground*

These days, as a citified mountain woman—a nature girl at heart—I sit here amid towering pine trees and inside a cabin with teas and tisanes. My pantry shelves are filled with boxes of tea varietals—and memories of when I was that twenty-something girl in Eugene, Oregon, who was envious of my host's tea collection and knowledge of tisanes. But now, I, too, have nature's gift and am gifted to understand the healing powers of tea.

These days, I intimately know specific teas and tisanes; they are like dear friends and family members—with different traits and healing powers—to help enhance my mind, body, and spirit. And now, I, and you, can differentiate which teas and tisanes to use for drinking, cooking, baking, and inside and outside of the household. No need to look at loose leaf tea with confusion. Those days are gone now that you've traveled along with me through the wonders of the land of tea.

I am inspired by the tea types and herbal varieties and the myriad of healing powers that are linked to each one. I confess that I do like the spicy varieties, such as cinnamon and orange spice, and the sweet and subtle flavor of white teas and bold, stronger black teas. The benefits of tea, from the amazing white tea beauty and bath products to soaps, pamper my body and spirit in the comfort of my home and when I travel, too.

MY JOURNEY THROUGH THE LAND OF TEA

What if I took another path in life and didn't experience hitching and hiking on the road buffered in the land of tea? What if I didn't struggle through the challenges of becoming a health author with tea to keep me balanced? What if I didn't like tea and drank alcohol like my blood relations? It took me decades to understand tea and its healing powers—and I'm still an apt tea pupil. Tea took care of me during times of poverty and abundance, during times of happiness and sadness, during times of love and loss. It was my muse, my energy, my solace, and it is my loyal friend forever.

For everything tea has taught me—I am grateful. My life—from childhood to adulthood and into my golden years—has included tea and tisanes in one form or type. Tea plays an integral role in who I am. How memorable it was on the road, how my life was enhanced with tea, like a best friend—then and now and in my future travels on the road and off at home.

Today in the 21st century there are doctors, nutritionists, and everyday people, maybe even you, who believe tea is a nice beverage—cold in the summer and hot in the winter. But if you have read this book from beginning to end, you understand that don't have to be a rocket scientist to know that tea is versatile, and is a special remedy. If you have doubts about the healing powers of tea, brew a cup of loose leaf tea—your favorite type—and please go back to chapter 1—or even to the end of each chapter and digest the highlights. I want you to get it. Tea is a gift that keeps on giving. Here, are a few tea tips I follow day to day.

Tea Tip 1: Listen to your body's cues. Turn to tea whether you're on top of the world or feeling a bit under the weather, like you do when you need a little help from a trustworthy friend or a companion animal.

Tea Tip 2: Eating whole natural foods like in the Oldways Mediterranean Diet Pyramid *and* pairing a variety of teas and tisanes to your daily regime will help you feel at your optimum best.

Tea Tip 3: Stay mindful while sipping tea. Living in the present (like the meditative monks who drank tea did) and knowing your purpose in life will help you feel focused and centered as well as help keep you young(er) and healthier for years to come.

So, as I come to the end of sharing *The Healing Powers of Tea* with you, while I haven't gone to tea gardens in Asia or tea estates in India, but I feel as if I have been there and back (and you can, too) when I brew, steep, and enjoy black, white, green, red teas—both commercial and specialty brands.

As you know, I have transformed from a toddler enjoying a tea party with imaginary guests and tea to a mature woman, a self-professed tea-aholic. I am in heaven while sitting in a tearoom in Vancouver, British Columbia, viewing a tea menu or roughing it on a nature tour in Seward, Alaska (eating berries, nuts, and seeds), and holding a thermos cup of plain black tea like my mother and her mother used to serve. Tea is a part of me, my spirit, and my soul.

The words of prime minister William Ewart Gladstone of the Victorian era say it best: "If you are cold, tea will warm you; if you are heated, it will cool you; if you are depressed, it will cheer you; if you are excited, it will calm you." And it's the powers of tea that take me to the special place I love—like home—and places in the heart. I am pleased to say with conviction and confidence, "It's tea time. Let me put the kettle on. How do you take your tea?"

PART 9

TEA
RESOURCES

Where Can You Buy Tea?

As tea continues to be touted for its powerful health benefits, quality tea for the health-conscious and specialty tea for serious tea enthusiasts (much like coffee and honey foodies), many are becoming more aware of this ancient superfood and its comeback around the globe. Currently, a wide world of teas can be bought in supermarkets, specialty stores, and health food stores, as well as through smaller tea companies on the Internet. And yes, the decision regarding which one is best can be subjective, just like when choosing your favorite olive oil and chocolate.

Here is a list of some teas and tea-infused products to help you widen your tea selection without traveling to another state or country. If you're interested in buying any of these popular tea or tea-related items, just contact the tea company directly for the locations of stores nearest you. Keep in mind, like any superfood, companies and people come and go, so if in the years to come, one of these establishments has expired like your favorite tea, please replace it with another. Change is unsettling but in the end it will be worth it so you can continue to enjoy your life in Tea World.

TOP-NOTCH RETAILERS

Here is a sampling of some of my favorite tea brands that are in my tea cupboard and in some of my own recipes in this book. Please note that tea companies can grow or merge with other companies, and are subject to change products.

Choice Organic Teas
790 Tennessee Street
San Francisco, CA 94107
http://www.choiceorganicteas.com

White teas, green teas, oolong teas, black teas, chai teas, and herbal teas.

Full Leaf Tea Company
2054 Antelope Road
White City, OR 97503
http://www.fullleafteacompany.com

Selected and curated the finest loose leaf tea and matcha from around the world.

Harney & Sons Fine Teas
5723 Route 22
Millerton, NY 12546
https://www.harney.com

An impressive assortment of teas and tisanes, beautiful packaging and presentation.

Mighty Leaf
100 Smith Ranch Road, Suite 120
San Rafael, CA 94903
www.mightyleaf.com

Specialty handcrafted tea blends.

Lipton Tea
www.liptontea.com

A global tea brand offering tea to 150 countries.

Numi
P.O. Box 20429
Oakland, CA 94620
www.numitea.com

Specializing in unique blends including green, black, white, and oolong teas.

R. C. Bigelow, Inc.
201 Black Rock Turnpike
Fairfield, CT 06825
www.bigelowtea.com

A famous American company sells a wide selection of teas and herbal teas.

Stash Tea
www.stashtea.com

Tea blends, tea gifts, treats and teaware, a variety of teas and herbal teas.

Special Tea Company
www.specialteacompany.com

Offers dozens of delicious specialty teas.

The Cozy Tea Cart
104A Route 13
Brookline, NH 03033
www.TheCozyTeaCart.com

Offers a wonderful selection of specialty teas.

SPECIALTY SHOPS
(CHOCOLATE, HERBAL TEA, OLIVE OIL, AND MORE)

MarieBelle New York
484 Broome Street
New York, NY 10013
www.mariebelle.com

A high-quality chocolate company offering tea-infused chocolate.

Vosges Haut-Chocolate
2950 North Oakley Avenue
Chicago, IL 60618
www.vosgeschocolate.com

A prestige chocolate company that provides chocolates infused with teas and spices.

Nick Sciabica & Sons
2150 Yosemite Boulevard
Modesto, CA 95354
www.sciabica.com

Specializes in olive oils using varieties of California olives. (See recipes created by Gemma Sciabica using their products.)

Wild Hibiscus Flower Company
www.wildhibiscus.com

Full range of innovative flower products includes flower teas.

TEA-RELATED ORGANIZATIONS

Tea and Herbal Association of Canada
133 Richmond Street West, Suite 207
Toronto, Ontario
www.tea.ca

The Tea Association of Canada supports the tea industry in the provinces and offers education about tea.

Tea Council of the U.S.A., Inc.
362 5th Avenue, Suite 801
New York, NY 10001
www.teausa.org

The Tea Council of the U.S.A. functions as the public and media relations component of the Tea Association of the U.S.A., Inc., and was established to support the promotion of tea in the U.S. Its recent focus has been almost exclusively on raising overall awareness of the science behind tea's health benefits, strengthened by the great taste, variety, and uniqueness of tea.

Specialty Tea Institute
362 5th Avenue, Suite 801
New York, NY 10001

The Specialty Tea Institute (STI) is the educational division of the Tea Association of the U.S.A., Inc., and the leader in the education of tea professionals.

HEALTH SPAS, TEA GARDENS, TEAROOMS, AND TEA SHOPS

Cal-a-Vie Health Spa
29402 Spa Havens Way
Vista, CA 92084
www.cal-a-vie.com

Japanese Tea Garden
75 Hagiwara Tea Garden Drive
San Francisco, CA 94102
http://www.japaneseteagardensf.com

Fairmont Hotel Vancouver
900 West Georgia Street
Vancouver British Columbia,
V6C 2W6, Canada
www.fairmont.com/hotel-vancouver/

Notes

CHAPTER 1:
THE POWER OF TEA

1. Patrick Donnelly, Melissa Stunk, Hueiwen Tan, Kunal Patel, Gabriel Agbor, Joe Vinson. Chemistry Department, University of Scranton, Scranton, PA. *Commercial Teas: Total Polyphenolic Antioxidant Content Using a New Hydrolysis and Isolation Procedure and Per Capita Contribution of Antioxidants.*
2. Liz Applegate, Ph.D. *101 Miracle Foods That Heal Your Heart* (New York: Prentice Hall, 2000), p. 267.
3. Jonny Bowden, Ph.D., C.N.S. *The 150 Healthiest Foods on Earth: The Surprising, Unbiased Truth About What You Should Eat and Why* (Beverly, MA: Fair Winds Press, 2007), p. 268.
4. Fatemeh Hajiaghaalipour, Junedah Sanusi, M. S. Kanthimathi. "Temperature and Time of Steeping Affect the Antioxidant Properties of White, Green, and Black Tea Infusions," *Journal of Food Science*, 2015; DOI: 10.1111/1750-3841.13149.
5. State of the U.S. Tea Industry Report 2015, by the Tea Association of the U.S.A., Inc.

CHAPTER 2:
AN ANCIENT CUPPA COMFORT

1. Babette Donaldson. *The Everything Healthy Tea Book: Discover the Healing Benefits of Tea* (Avon, MA: Adams Media, 2014), p. 34.
2. Ibid., p. 36.
3. Tea Fact Sheet–2015. Tea Association of the U.S.A., Inc.
4. Ibid.
5. Sarah Begley. "A Brief History of the Tea Bag," September 3, 2015; time.com/a-brief-history-of-the-tea-bag. (Accessed June 6, 2016.)
6. Caroline Dow. *The Healing Powers of Tea: Simple Teas & Tisanes to Remedy and Rejuvenate Your Health* (Woodbury, MN: Llewellyn Publications, 2014), p. 3.
7. Babette Donaldson. *The Everything Healthy Tea Book: Discover the Healing Benefits of Tea* (Avon, MA: Adams Media, 2014), p. 39.

CHAPTER 4:
NOTEWORTHY NUTRIENTS

1. Kijoon Kim, Terrence M. Vance, Ock K. Chun. "Estimated intake and major food sources of flavonoids among U.S. adults: changes between 1999–2002 and 2007–2010 in NHANES," *Eur J Nutr* (2016) 55:833-843 DOI 10. 1007/s00394-015-0942-x.

CHAPTER 5:
BLACK TEA, YOU'RE AMAZING!

1. Tea & Health: An Overview of Research on the Potential Health Benefits of Tea. Tea U.S.A.
2. I. Dora, L. Arab, A. Martinchik, A. Sdvizhkov, L. Urbanovich, U. Weisgerber. "Black tea consumption and risk of rectal cancer in Moscow population," *Ann Epidemiol*, 2003 Jul; 13 (6): 405–11.
3. Health Council of the Netherlands. Dutch dietary guidelines 2015. The Hague: Health Council of the Netherlands, 2015; publication no. 2015/24E. ISBN 978-94-6281-104-1.
4. Ariel Beresniak, Gerard Duru, Genevieve Berger, Dominique Bremond-Gignac. "Relationships between black tea consumption

and key health indicators in the world: an ecological study," *BMJ* 2012:2 e00068 doi:10.1136.

5. Tea U.S.A. Heart Health 11–15 Tea Association of the U.S.A., Inc.

6. Jonny Bowden. *The 150 Healthiest Foods on Earth: The Surprising, Unbiased Truth about What You Should Eat and Why* (Beverly, MA: Fair Winds Press, 2007), p. 266.

7. S. C. Laren, J. Virtamo, A. Wolk. "Black tea consumption and risk of stroke in women and men," *Ann Epidemiol.* 2013 Mr; 23(3):157–60.

8. D. Grassi, G. Desideri, P. Di Giosia, M. De Feo, E. Fellini, P. Cheli, L. Ferri, C. Ferri. "Tea, flavonoids, and cardiovascular health: endotheial protection," *Am J Clin Nutr.* 2013 De; 98 (Suppl): 1660S–1666S. [Epub 2013 Oct 30].

CHAPTER 6:
THE WHITE TEA REVOLUTION

1. Babette Donaldson. *The Everything Healthy Tea Book: Discovering the Healing Benefits of Tea* (Avon, MA: Adams Media, 2014), p. 152.

CHAPTER 7:
THE OLD AND NEW INCREDIBLE INGREDIENTS

1. Mark Ukra, Sharon Kolberg. *The Ultimate Tea Diet: How Tea Can Boost Your Metabolism, Shrink Your Appetite, and Kick-Start Remarkable Weight Loss* (New York: William Morrow, 2007), p. 15.

2. Gian Carlo Tenore, Pietrol Campiglia, Daniela Giannetti, Novellino, Ettore. "Simulated gastrointestinal digestion, intestinal permeation and plasma protein interaction of white, green, and black tea polyphenols," *Food Chemistry* 169 (2015), pp. 320–326.

CHAPTER 8:
IS WHITE TEA GOOD FOR YOU?

1. Tamsyn Thring, Pauline Hili, and Declan P. Naughton. "Anti-collagenase, anti-elastase and anti-oxidant activities of extracts from

21 plants," *BMC Complementary and Alternative Medicine.* (ISCMR)20099:27 DOI: 10.1186/1472-6882-9-27.
2. Mark Ukra, Sharon Kolberg. *The Ultimate Tea Diet: How Tea Can Boost Your Metabolism, Shrink Your Appetite, and Kick-Start Remarkable Weight Loss* (New York: William Morrow: 2007), p. 15.
3. Tamsyn Thring, Pauline Hili, and Declan P. Naughton. "Anti-collagenase, anti-elastase and anti-oxidant activities of extracts from 21 plants," *BMC Complementary and Alternative Medicine.* (ISCMR) 20099:27 DOI: 10.1186/1472-6882-9-27.

CHAPTER 9:
HEALTHY GREEN TEA

1. Shengmin Sang, Joshua D. Lambert, Chi-Tang Ho, Chung S. Yang. "The chemistry and biotransformation of tea constituents," *Pharmacol Res.* 2011;64(2):87–99.
2. S. Kuriyama, T. Shirnazu, K. Ohmori, N. Kikuchi, N. Nakaya, Y. Nishino, Y. Tsubono, I. Tsuji. "Green tea consumption and mortality due to cardiovascular disease, cancer, and all causes in Japan: the Ohsaki study." JAMA. 2006 Sep 13;296(10):1255–65.

CHAPTER 10:
THE RED TEA BOOM

1. Jonny Bowden, Ph.D., C.N.S. *The 150 Healthiest Foods on Earth: The Surprising, Unbiased Truth About What You Should Eat and Why* (Beverly, MA: Fair Winds Press, 2007), p. 264.
2. Cal Orey, *101 Doctors: What Doctors Do to Stay Healthy* (New York: Kensington Publishing, 2002), pp. 83, 85, 95.

CHAPTER 11:
HEALING HERBAL TEAS

1. B. T. Howrey, K. S. Markides, J. M. McKee, et al. "Chamomile Consumption and Mortality: A Prospective Study of Mexican Origin Older Adults," *The Gerontologist*, 2015, doi: 10. 1093geront/gnv051.

CHAPTER 12:
TEA(S) MEDITERRANEAN-STYLE

1. Cecilia Samieri, Ph.D., et. al. "The Association Between Dietary Patterns at Midlife and Health in Aging: An Observational Study," *Ann Intern Med.* 2013; I 159 (9): 584–591.

CHAPTER 13:
THE SKINNY ON TEA AND FAT

1. R. An, J. McCaffrey. "Plain water consumption in relation to energy intake and diet quality among US adults, 2005–2012," *Journal of Human Nutrition and Dietetics.* March 1, 2016; DOI:10.1111/jhn.12368.

CHAPTER 14:
AGE-DEFYING DREAM POTION

1. C. L. Shen, M. C. Chyu, J. Wang. "Tea and bone health: steps forward in translational nutrition," *Am J Clin Nutr,* 2013 Dec. 98 (6 Suppl): 1694S–1699S.
2. S. A. Tamsyn, Pauline Hili Thring, Declan P. Naughton. "Anti-collagenase, anti-elastase and anti-oxidant activities of extracts from 21 plants," *BMC Complementary and Alternative Medicine,* 2009, 9:27 (4 August 2009); DOI: 10.1186/1472-6882-9-27.
3. American Heart Association's Epidemiology/Lifestyle 2016 Scientific Sessions. American Heart Association News. (Retrieved March 1, 2016. EPI 2016 news stories.)

CHAPTER 15:
HOME REMEDIES FROM YOUR KITCHEN

1. The editors of FC&A Medical Publishing. *The Folk Remedy Encyclopedia: Olive Oil, Vinegar, Honey and 1,001 Other Home Remedies* (Peachtree City, GA: Frank W. Cawood and Associates, Inc., 2004), p. 9.

2. Fabian Fernandex, Jamie O. Edgin."Pharmacotherapy in Down's syndrome: which way forward?" *Lancet Neurol.* 2016, DOI: (16) 30056-4).

3. The editors of FC&A Medical Publishing. *The Folk Remedy Encyclopedia: Olive Oil, Vinegar, Honey and 1,001 Other Home Remedies* (Peachtree City, GA: Frank W. Cawood and Associates, Inc., 2004), p. 210.

4. M. Kushiyama, Y. Shimazaki, M. Murakami, Yamashita. "Relationship between intake of green tea and periodontal disease," *J Periodontal*, Mar 2009, 80 (3):32–7.

5. B. Nugala, A. Namasi, P. Emmadi, P. M. Krishna. "Role of green tea and periodontal disease. The Asian paradox," *J Indian Soc Periodontol* 2012 Jul–Sep; 16(3):313–316.

6. G. C. Curhan, W. C. Willett, E. B. Rimm, D. Spiegelman, M. J. Stampfer. "Prospective study of beverage use and the risk of kidney stones," *Am J Epidemiol* 1996; 143:240–7.

7. E. L. Gibson, R. Vounonvirta, et al. "The effects of tea on psychophysiological stress responsivity and post-stress recovery," *The Journal of Psychopharmacology* (2007) 190: 81. doi:10.1007/s00213-006-0573-2.

CHAPTER 18:
NOT EVERYONE'S CUP OF TEA

1. The International Agency for Research on Cancer Monograph Working Group. "Carcinogenicity of drinking coffee, mate, and very hot beverages," *The Lancet Oncology*, published online June 15, 2016.

Selected Bibliography

Arndorfer, Travis, and Kristine Hansen. *The Complete Idiot's Guide to Coffee & Tea*. New York: Alpha Books, 2006.

Bowden, Jonny, Ph.D., C.N.S. *The 150 Healthiest Foods on Earth: The Surprising, Unbiased Truth About What You Should Eat and Why*. Beverly, MA: Fair Winds Press, 2007.

Donaldson, Babette. *The Everything Healthy Tea Book: Discover the Healing Benefits of Tea*. Avon, MA: Adams Media, 2014.

Dow, Caroline. *The Healing Power of Tea: Simple Teas & Tisanes to Remedy and Rejuvenate Your Health*. Woodbury, MN: Llewellyn Publications, 2014.

Gasoyne, Francoiz Marchand, Jasmin Desharnais, and Hugo Americi. *Tea: History Terroirs Varieties*, Second Edition, The Camellia Sinesis Tea House. Buffalo, NY: A Firefly Book, 2014.

Harvest House Publishers. *365 Things Every Tea Lover Should Know*. Eugene, OR: Harvest House Publishers, 2008.

Safi, Tammy. *Healthy Teas. Green-Black-Herbal-Fruit*: Hong Kong, China: Periplus Editions, 2001.

Sciabica, Gemma Sanita. *Baking Sensational Sweets and California Olive Oil*. Modesto, CA: Gemma Sanita Sciabica, 2005.

Sciabica, Gemma Sanita. *Baking with California Olive Oil: Dolci and Biscotti Recipes*. Modesto, CA: Gemma Sanita Sciabica, 2002.

Sciabica, Gemma Sanita. *Cooking with California Olive Oil: Popular Recipes*. Modesto, CA: Gemma Sanita Sciabica, 2001.

Sciabica, Gemma Sciabica. *Cooking with California Olive Oil: Recipes from the Heart for the Heart:* Modesto, CA: Gemma Sanita Sciabica, 2009.

Sciabica, Gemma Sanita. *Cooking with California Olive Oil: Treasured Family Recipes.* Modesto, CA: Gemma Sanita Sciabica, 1998.

Connect with Us

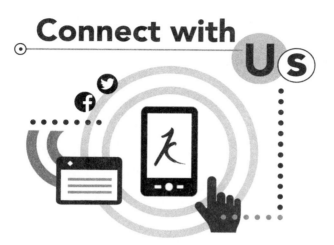

Visit us online at
KensingtonBooks.com
to read more from your favorite authors, see books
by series, view reading group guides, and more.

for sneak peeks, chances to win books and prize packs,
and to share your thoughts with other readers.

facebook.com/kensingtonpublishing
twitter.com/kensingtonbooks

Tell us what you think!

To share your thoughts, submit a review,
or sign up for our eNewsletters, please visit:
KensingtonBooks.com/TellUs.